A SCEPTIC'S MEDICAL DICTIONARY

D0774694

For my postgraduate tutors Sharon Banoff, Joy Hatwood, Chris Paling, Michael Milan, and the Dog Chairman.

Also by Michael O'Donnell:
The devil's prison
An insider's guide to the games doctors play
The long walk home
How to succeed in business without sacrificing your health

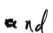 with much love

Michael

A SCEPTIC'S MEDICAL DICTIONARY

Michael O'Donnell

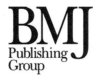

BMJ
Publishing
Group

The right of Michael O'Donnell to be identified as the author of this work has been
asserted by him in accordance with the Copyright, Designs and Patents Act 1988.

First published in 1997
by the BMJ Publishing Group, BMA House, Tavistock Square,
London WC1H 9JR

British Library Cataloguing in Publication Data

A catalogue record for this book is available
from the British Library

ISBN 0-7279-1204-6

The figure on the front cover is based on the Lincoln Imp, a 13th century stone carving
in Lincoln Cathedral.

Typeset by Apek Typesetters Ltd, Nailsea, Bristol
Printed and bound in Great Britain by Latimer Trend, Plymouth

Sceptic

One who suspects the world would be a healthier place if fewer people had the courage of their convictions and more had the courage of their doubts.

I never submitted the whole system of my opinions to the creed of any party of men whatever, in religion, in philosophy, in politics or in anything else, where I was capable of thinking for myself. Such an addiction is the last degradation of a free and moral agent. If I could not go to Heaven but with a party, I would not go there at all.

Thomas Jefferson

Aaronical

A high priestly, pontifical role that some doctors think appropriate for their profession. Correct spelling: Ironical.

> What the public and we are inclined to forget is that doctors are different. We establish standards of professional conduct. This is where we differ from the rag, tag, and bobtail crew who like to think of themselves as professionals in the health field.
> *Paul Vickers, consultant surgeon and General Medical Councillor, addressing a BMA meeting in 1978. Three years later he was found guilty of murdering his wife with an anticancer drug*

> Doctors are not gods, and function best as loyal, devoted, skilful servants, advising, persuading, supporting, but never usurping. The best doctor is a kind of Jeeves.
> Donald Gould. *The Black and White Medicine Show*, Hamish Hamilton, 1985

Academy of Medicine

A fantasy that afflicts doctors of a certain age as inevitably as the symptoms of prostatic obstruction.

> As distinguished men approach the end of their careers, many are struck by the need for a comfortable institution, built above a well-stocked cellar, where wise men such as themselves—and maybe a carefully selected handful of women—could reflect upon the activities of those who are actually doing the work and issue declarations on the great moral and ethical dilemmas of our time.
> Anecdotal evidence. *Healthcare Management*, January 1995

> The Loch Ness monster of medicine. Sometimes you see it; sometimes you don't. It disappears for decades and then pops up again through the mist in all kinds of fuzzy, indefinable shapes. It is protean, ageless, grotesque, and fascinating, all at the same time. To those of us with an addiction to freaks and fancies it is irresistible. The proposal for an Academy of Medicine resurfaced on March 24, 1973, in the *BMJ*, after having been peacefully submerged for almost a quarter of a century...

It would, according to its sponsors, be a forum for discussion and a medium for collaboration. It would present a united voice on matters of special concern. In fact it would be just another committee of eminent gentlemen, without either authority or the strength that comes from democratic representation. As an institution, it would be so bland and innocuous as to be hardly visible at all.

John Rowan Wilson. *World Medicine*, 4 April 1973

Accountants

People of a particular cast of mind, not necessarily trained in accountancy. As in: "During the 1990s, accountants took over the NHS and the BBC". *See* Grey Suits.

The most insidious legacy of Thatcherism [is] its comprehensive implementation of the proposition that the only views which matter are those of men (they are mostly men) in suits who spend their lives crawling along the "bottom line". Everywhere we look—broadcasting, the arts, universities, the health service, research councils, quangos of every ilk—we find courts and councils and boards of governors and trustees stuffed with accountants, company directors, management consultants and other proponents of commercial realism.

Don't get me wrong. I have nothing against businessmen....They are, after all, members of the public and as such should be represented on public bodies. All I object to is the attitude that they are the only people whose views really count.

John Naughton. Crawling along the bottom line. *Observer*,
7 January 1996

In the same way that patients have become an inconvenience to the profitability of the NHS trust, broadcasting has become a rather strange exhaust thrown out of the back of a machine which is doing serious bureaucratic work.

Interview with Jonathan Miller. *Daily Telegraph*,
9 September 1995

Acronyms

Word game that medical organisations play with an enthusiasm outmatched only by NASA and the Pentagon.

I first noticed the burgeoning obsession with acronyms with the coming of ASH, an organisation whose objectives win my passionate approval yet whose title "Action on Smoking and Health" seems to overstrain syntax to achieve acronymic status. The condition is infectious. The creation of ASH caused the tobacco lobby to fight back with FOREST and the doctors to respond, dare I say equally woodenly, with TREES.

One man's burden. *BMJ*, 13 September 1986

The most noticeable additives to the British diet over the past few years have been acronyms, and those who don't take an obsessional interest in such things may need a guide. As well as COMA, the Committee on Medical Aspects of Food Policy, there is JACNE, the Joint Advisory Committee on Nutrition Education, which replaced NACNE, the National Advisory Committee, etc, etc. The word national in NACNE is said to have been added because of the unacceptability of the acronym without it.

One man's burden. *BMJ*, 26 October 1985

NATASHA is the new acronym for the National Truss and Surgical Appliance Society, founded in 1772 by William Pitt and originally known as "An Institute for Relief of the Ruptured Poor".

Looking sideways. *Medical Monitor*, 18 October 1991

News reaches me that the South Carolina Organisation of Ophthalmological Practitioners is not best pleased that its acronym SCOOP has been hijacked by a New York campaign to prevent dogs from defecating in the streets. In New York, it seems, the initials stand not for all that's best in ophthalmology but for Stop Crapping On Our Pavements.

Medical Monitor, 8 September 1993

Added value

What customers, once known as patients, really want from the NHS.

Success in marketing clinical services to "customers", rather than the ability to cure them, should become the benchmark for judging NHS performance.

That, says the *Independent*, was the view of Dr Mark Baker, the Bradford Hospital Trust's chief executive when, earlier this month, he exhorted a conference of health service managers to "hail successful selling staff as the heroes of the organisation".

Other staff, he said, needed to manage their time more efficiently. Patients received "value" for only about 5% of the time they were in contact with the service.

Looking sideways. *Medical Monitor*, 20 September 1991

Dr Baker's observation supports results from a recent study of GPs' work load carried out by several high minded persons, including myself.

We discovered that 68.9% of GPs waste valuable NHS time shaking hands with their customers as they enter or leave the surgery. And that a shocking 89.6% waste time talking to customers about things that have nothing to do with their illness, like the weather, gardening, football, news of their families, or local gossip.

Ibid

Aggressive dysarthria

A way of turning a disability to advantage.

Patrick Campbell was not the only Irishman who could manipulate a stutter. Some years ago I had dinner in Dublin with a judge whose home was regularly picketed by political demonstrators. Most times the picketing was reasonably good humoured but one day a more aggressive mob than usual marched up the drive.

As they approached the house, they were confronted by the judge's bodyguard, a gun-toting but stuttering police sergeant.

"S-s-s-stand right where you are", said the sergeant. "If one of you f-f-f-f-effers comes a s-s-s-step nearer, I'll blow his f-f-f-f-ing head off".

"Don't swear at these representatives of the people", said the leader of the mob.

"With this s-s-s-s-stutter", said the sergeant, "I can't f-f-f-f-fing swear".

Medical Monitor, 22 January 1993

Alternative medicines

Remedies that are neither medicines nor alternative. Officially marketed as food supplements to avoid the provisions of the Medicines Act. Sales patter makes great play with words like **natural** and **holistic**.

Favourite elixirs of the decade included Royal Jelly— "Nature's richest health food", an extract from the sexual organs of New Zealand mussels, and the more scientifically pretentious Spagyrik therapy which claims to cure "practically all illnesses". Spagyrik suffered little loss of credibility when two of its directors acknowledged that their Doctor of Science degrees were awarded by the International University of Sri Lanka which, though unrecognised in Sri Lanka, meets from time to time on holiday in Malaga.

The decade opened with a comeback by ginseng, a humble tuber whose reputation for potency derives from its anatomical resemblance to the male sexual apparatus, and closed with emergency warnings from the Department of Health about the dangers of two health food ingredients, germanium and L-tryptophan.

An unhealthy pursuit of the unobtainable. *Daily Telegraph*,
19 December 1989

Annenberg syndrome

Speech impediment that occurs when self importance determines a speaker's vocabulary and syntax. Named after Walter Annenberg, one time American Ambassador to London. Television cameras present at his first meeting with the Queen recorded his reply when she asked him how he was settling into the embassy.

Your majesty will not be cognisant with the fact that at this point in actuality...we have unscheduled logistical and transportation deferments...so that predicted levels of refurbishment items ... why, er, at this time we have a shortfall in our present, er, what we would normally, er, acceptable refurbishment levels.

Royal Family. BBC Television 1969

These outbursts of fluent Martian are generated by an

5

Obfuscation Centre which is less likely to lie in the cortex than close to the anal sphincter. Outbreaks had been reported before Annenberg made his definitive utterance.
In the 1960s a Pentagon official briefed the press on the tactical advantages of the neutron bomb in these words: "The egress of neutrons from a low energy burst has the primary effect of dislocation of biological function at cellular level whilst leaving macro-inorganic structures undamaged".
To which a reporter from the *Denver Post* responded: "Yeah, well, that's fine if you're a front porch".
Dr Rod Manton, Associate Adviser in General Practice to the North West Region. *Personal communication*

Pseudo-Annenberg Syndrome

The use of obfuscation not to sustain self importance but to insulate speaker and audience from the meaning of what is being said.

We are not running a two tier system. We are merely prioritising our admission protocols on the basis of different parameters.
Hospital Trust chairman replying to critic at public meeting,
1994

Arts, The

Source of wisdom ignored by medical **educationalists**.

The things that really matter to us—the secrets of the heart, of what it means to be an individual, the depths and heights of human experience—all are accessible, if at all, only through literature and the creative arts. Science has no purchase on them, and precious little to say about them beyond the posturings of reductionists. A knowledge of the biochemistry of the brain tells us nothing about the mind of its owner. And even when the whole of the human genome has been mapped, we will still not know what makes us tick.
John Naughton. Notes on life, liberty and the pursuit of power. *Observer,* 9 July 1995

We feel that even when all possible scientific questions have been answered, the problems of life remain completely unanswered.
Ludwig Wittgenstein.
In: Hugh Whitmore, *Breaking the Code*, Amber Lane Press
1986

One of the things the average doctor doesn't have time to do is catch up with the things he didn't learn in school, and one of the things he didn't learn in school is the nature of human society, its purpose, its history, and its needs....If medicine is necessarily a mystery to the average man, nearly everything else is necessarily a mystery to the average doctor.
Milton Mayer. *Monitor Weekly*, 26 January 1994

Aspirational dyscrasia

Two disorders of articulation. As resistant to treatment as **irritable vowel syndrome**.

Itinerant aspirate
Condition in which aspirates migrate from one word to another. Mistakenly thought to afflict only northerners

> The disorder also occurs in Bedfordshire. Jim Aylward, a GP in Ampthill has a patient who, when asked his first name, always replies "'Orace with a Haitch". And another recently opened the batting in a consultation by saying: "Sorry to trouble you doctor but I've got a problem with my harse".
> The itinerant aspirate has been built into some fine old Bedfordshire sayings. Yet another of Dr Aylward's patients ended her lively description of uncontrollable lower bowel turbulence with the remark: "As my old mother used to say, doctor, it's a sad harse that never laughs".
> *Medical Monitor*, 15 May 1966

Showering aspirate
Less common than the itinerant form. Occurs in people who can switch off sibilant sounds only by inserting an aspirate, making them sound as if they are talking through loose false teeth. One well known sufferer is Lord Deedes, former editor of the *Daily*

7

Telegraph and occasional parenthetic intervener in *Private Eye*: ("shurely shome mishtake").

I always thought the showering aspirate occurred only in speech. But recently Dr F W D Debney found one in a caption in the Abingdon Herald: "The Saxton Road Playgroup is shown receiving a tree, one of the first offered by the Vale of White Horse District Council as part of their campaign to Shit in the Shade".

Medical Monitor, 12 June 1996

Astrology

The only "science" editors of British newspapers and television current affairs programmes seem to understand.

When the BBC started breakfast television, we could, if we got up early enough on a Thursday morning, get a word of advice from a doctor. We had less difficulty catching the resident astrologer who appeared every day predicting the future with a dogmatic certainty that the poor quack, tethered by reason, could never hope to match.

Body and soul. *Guardian*, August 1984

A Bristol magazine *The Grapevine* recently carried a full page article by an astrologer who can "predict health patterns from the constellations". The author is not one of your cheapskate, common or garden astrologers but a "medical astrologer".

Did you know that Pluto is a trigger planet and governs illnesses that either "disrupt the body like cancer or develop progressively like multiple sclerosis or ME?" Did you know that "the brain can't operate without Uranus?"...Or that when the Moon, Neptune, and Saturn get into a particular relationship this "could trigger stomach cancer?"...

Given that the article is headed "Preventative Medicine" the author is strangely silent about what his readers can actually do to keep the planets in line and prevent these terrible things happening.

Healthwatch Newsletter, May 1995

Dr Shawn Carlson of the University of California carried out two exhaustive investigations of astrological inter-pretations conducted with the cooperation of astrologers highly regarded within their trade. After three years' investigation, he concluded: "Despite the fact that we worked with some of the best astrologers...despite the fact they approved of the design of the experiment and predicted 50% as the minimum effect they would expect to see, astrology failed to perform at a level better than chance".

That sort of evidence suggests to doctors that astrology is unlikely to be of much use to their patients except as an entertaining source of after dinner conversation. Medical science has the marginal advantage of being based on a system of logic. After all, television producers in search of weather forecasts still rely on those dear old meteorologists, despite their failings. They don't get the newscaster to disembowel an animal and give us a read of the entrails. Nor show some old salt having a feel of his seaweed.

The medical condition. *The Listener*, 12 May 1988

Audiogenic confusion

Common interpretative dysfunction. Most people hear only what they want to hear.

A medical student doing a holiday job as a dogsbody at a regional health authority was asked to deliver a package to a Mr Ernest Sexhauer. Not knowing where to find him, he rang the telephonist at the nearest district hospital.

"Do you have a Sexhauer there?" he asked.

"No", she replied. "We don't even have a ten minute coffee break".

Anecdotal evidence. *Healthcare Management*, March 1993

A correspondent told me that as a child she was for a long time confused about the part played in the Anglican communion by a fabulous beast called the Prairie Tortoise. At some point in the service, at Sunday school or school assembly, the congregation would cry out excitedly, "Let us hear the Prairie Tortoise", and my correspondent says she always hoped that the creature's characteristic whinny might somehow be reproduced. A long time afterwards, running the phrase through her head, she realised there was no such animal, just a pious hope to hear the prayer he taught us. My friend Skinner adds that he often wondered why the service took such a personal turn when the whole congregation would kneel down and groan, "Pray for us Skinners"— though, he said, he knew the family stood in more than ordinary need of it.

Robert Robinson. *The Dog Chairman*, Allen Lane, 1982

Margaret Barker, a consultant paediatrician in Dorchester, found a page in the March edition of *The Sarum Link* dominated by the headline: "Harvest of the Sewers". She read the article beneath expecting to learn of some new biological method of reclaiming valuable essences from effluent but discovered that the story was about a group of dedicated embroiderers who were replacing shabby hassocks in Salisbury Cathedral.

Anecdotal evidence. *Medical Interface*, May 1996

Autocratic Perseverance Syndrome

Sometimes known as the Lady Bracknell diathesis. Confusional state induced by attempts to correct those who know everything.

The playwright Michael Frayn was approached at the BAFTA awards by a man who said: "I very much enjoyed your play about Joe Egg". Frayn explained politely that the play was written by Peter Nichols and that the pair were often confused.

"Oh no", said the man emphatically, "I know Frayn and I'm talking about your play". The gentle Frayn turned his attention elsewhere but some months later at another party found himself alongside the same man.

"Do you remember when we met at the BAFTA awards", said Frayn, "You confused me with Peter Nichols?" The man stared at him sternly and barked: "I've never been to the BAFTA awards".

Medical Monitor, 11 December 1996

A gentler form of the syndrome was reported in *Hospital Doctor* by Dr M A A Rahman, a research fellow in rheumatology at London's University College Hospital. Some years ago a patient he describes as "a charming lady" told him proudly that her abdominal scar was the relic of a hysterectomy performed by Sir Geoffrey Howe.

Noting Dr Rahman's reaction she said: "Oh, I'm sorry, have I made a mistake? Is he not a Sir?"

"It's not that", said the good doctor. "It's just that Sir

Geoffrey Howe is Chancellor of the Exchequer".
The charming lady beamed back. "Fancy that. Hasn't he
done well?"

Ibid

———— •◆◆• ————

Back-up services

(Obsolete) Mutual support that hospital departments once offered
each another.
(Now) Methods of extracting additional revenue from patients.

Jean Clark went into the Princess Royal Hospital in
Haywards Heath last week for an internal stomach examination. While Mrs Clark was recovering, a member of the
hospital staff dropped by to ask if she might like a video of
the endoscopy for £10.
Matthew Norman. *Guardian*, 27 July 1995

"It is a simple medical fact that to sustain a high quality, safe
accident and emergency service requires a large department
with a full range of back-up services", said Tom Sackville,
the junior Health Minister.
   The Royal London is the new face of London's accident
and emergency provision of which Mr Sackville is so
immeasurably proud. In the main waiting room, a video
monitor entertains waiting casualties with the latest news,
star sign analysis ("Leo, you may have cause to take
medical advice this week") and advertisements ("Benji's
Nite spot: Nurses come free!"). You can pass the time in W
H Smith, browsing magazines, or buy sandwiches from the
internal market operating in the foyer. The wait, however,
remains the same. And, according to senior doctors, the
chances of receiving appropriate care have significantly
declined.
News report. *Independent*, 27 January 1995

Bacon, Francis

Elizabethan philosopher who, when not writing Shakespeare's
plays, suggested that if man could collect all the information that

was available about the world he would completely understand it. Still exerts an unhealthy influence on medicine. *See* Galileo.

> During its journey from mystic certainty towards scientific uncertainty, medicine has never quite shrugged off its faith in the inductive approach of Francis Bacon
> ...It's remarkable how many doctors still seem to think that the way to apply science to medicine is to act like a vacuum cleaner, collecting vast quantities of data, all carefully observed and punctiliously recorded. Yet as Peter Medawar wrote while he was director of the MRC: "Sciences which remain at Bacon's level of development... amount to little more than academic play".
> And William Harvey, who was Bacon's doctor, said of his patient: "He writes philosophy like a Lord Chancellor".
> The toxic effect of language on medicine.
> *Journal of the Royal College of Physicians of London*, November/December 1995

> Where is the understanding we have lost in knowledge?
> Where is the knowledge we have lost in information?
> T S Elliot. Choruses from The Rock.
> In: *Collected poems 1909-1962*, Faber

Beans-in-a-jar hypothesis

If you put a bean in a jar for each coition in the first year of a marriage, and remove a bean from the jar for each coition in subsequent years, you will never empty the jar. *See* de Vries effect.

Bed shortage

Myth perpetuated by nurses and doctors to embarrass politicians who know that the NHS's problem is not too few but too many beds.

> A six year old girl has been denied vital heart surgery for the third time because of a shortage of hospital beds. Jemma Evans's latest disappointment came after she had been given "pre-op" medication and was about to taken into the

operating theatre. After nurses at Birmingham Children's Hospital removed the drip tubes from her arms, she was taken home in tears. This was the third postponement she had endured.

Paul Stokes. *Daily Telegraph*, 5 August 1995

Bedside manner

Medical salesmanship. There are three traditional approaches.

• Charm or sympathy "switched on" as a deliberate technique rather than generated by genuine empathy. Sometimes called the "game show host" approach. *See* Communication skills. Not particularly reassuring to patients.

• Impressive self confidence born of ignorance and lack of insight. Most common in specialists in diseases of the rich. Highly reassuring to patients, even those of some intelligence.

In a stage direction in *The Doctor's Dilemma* George Bernard Shaw describes how the bombastic Sir Ralph Bloomfield Bonnington cheers, reassures and heals his patients because anxiety and disease are incompatible with his commanding presence. "Even broken bones, it is said, have been known to unite at the sound of his voice".

Medical Monitor, May 1997

• A quiet and caring air that gives each patient the impression that he or she is the only person on the doctor's mind. Can be the most reassuring manner of all.

In the 1930s and '40s, a GP in Cork, who was always referred to as Doctor Kearney, as if Doctor were his first name, would say to the relatives of a sick man: "We'll be a little bit worried about him for the next 24 hours".

It left the relatives with a reassuring image of the kindly doctor going about his business the next day with part of his mind constantly concerned about the health of their loved one.

And whatever the outcome, the doctor appeared to have anticipated it. If the patient took a turn for the worse, the relatives said to themselves: "The doctor gave us a hint of what might happen but was kind enough to break it gently".

And if the patient recovered, as patients have a tendency to do despite the most rigorous of treatment, the doctor's 24

hours of concern was seen, in some mysterious way, to have played a part in the recovery.
Monitor Weekly, 21 September 1994

Belgrano

New name for Guy's Hospital: the flagship that moved in the wrong direction and got sunk.

Berlin Wall

One of the less well publicised ingredients of homeopathic remedies.

This patient continues to have multiple symptoms of lumps on scalp and has had a flu-like illness. Overall her mood has improved, however, I have given her a dose of Carcinosin Nosode 30c over the day followed by Berlin Wall 30c once a day in the morning...
Letter from Royal London Homeopathic Hospital to London GP, Cornel Fleming, August 1996

What therapeutic advantages does Berlin Wall have over ordinary garden wall or Spaghetti Junction concrete? And do Scottish homeopaths use microdoses of that historic nostrum, Hadrian's Wall? I think we should be told.
Medical Monitor, 18 September 1996

Best type of general practice

That which doctors, rather than their patients, prefer: large groups, comprehensive clinical services, multidisciplinary teams, etc.

This study shows that patients prefer a personal service. Given the current approach to practice organisation, patients are more likely to obtain a service that meets their requirements if they attend small, non-training practices that operate personal list systems.
Richard Baker, Jane Streatfield. What type of practice do patients prefer? *Journal of the Royal College of General Practitioners*, December 1995

Blame

Something that someone has to shoulder after any mishap.

Declining faith in the existence of God prevents misfortune from being attributed to His will. Increasing faith in the benevolence of all things natural prevents acceptance of natural catastrophes. The notion of bad luck is applied only to picking the wrong numbers in the National Lottery.

Medical Monitor, 18 October 1995

I take it as axiomatic that all men want to be free: free, that is, of the consequences of their own actions. When things go well, they praise themselves; when they go badly, they call a doctor. The function of the doctor is to furnish excuses, whether to wives or to courts.

Theodore Dalrymple.
If Symptoms Persist, Andre Deutsch, 1994

Mistakes are at the very base of human thought, embedded there, feeding the structure like root nodules. If we were not provided with the knack of being wrong, we could never get anything useful done. We think our way along by choosing between right and wrong alternatives, and the wrong choices have to be made as frequently as the right ones.

We get along in life this way. We are built to make mistakes, coded for error. We learn, as we say, by "trial and error". Why do we always say that? Why not "trial and rightness" or "trial and triumph"? The old phrase puts it that way because that is, in real life, the way it is done.

Lewis Thomas.
The Medusa and the Snail, Viking Press, 1976

Blonde

Sultry siren in a "Top Doc Sex Shock". *See* Dirty docs.

MRC sociologists who surveyed newspaper coverage of GMC disciplinary hearings found that the tabloids almost always described the "other woman" as a blonde. During the hearing, the wronged wife was dark haired and "prim and proper". After the hearing she was "devoted and loving'" if the doctor was found not guilty; "loyal" or "standing by her man" if he was struck off.

The relationship between "blonde" and hair colour seemed arbitrary. One blonde in the *Daily Express* and *Daily Mail* was a brunette in the *News Of The World*. A blonde in the *Daily Mirror* was auburn haired in the *Daily Mail*.

Medical Monitor, 5 March 1997

Blood cholesterol

Biochemical measurement that some men, many of them American, treat as a golfer treats his handicap: working on it, taking pride in its reduction, and introducing it, none too artfully, into conversation.

BMAspeak

Coded language used by BMA politicians at their Annual Representative Meeting. Compare **obituary prose**.

> This is surely a matter of principle:
> This involves money.
> This is a matter of high principle:
> This involves a lot of money.
> Those of us who are in real contact with patients:
> The General Medical Services (GMS) committee.
> The profession at large:
> The GMS committee.
> The people of these islands:
> The GMS committee.
> Our general practice colleagues:
> That blackguard of a GP whose name I can never remember.
> Our friend from the regions:
> That unspeakable hick whose name I certainly won't admit to knowing.
> Our valued delegate from the junior staff:
> That sickening young upstart whose name I have carefully noted.
> I am sorry to have to challenge the accuracy of para 147 of the Minutes:
> Para 147 is an accurate account of the committee's having once again failed to appreciate my point of view.

On a point of order:
  In the hope of prolonging the present disorder.
We're always grateful for a breath of fresh Northern air:
  Those bloody Scots.
I take the point:
  What a load of rubbish.
A valuable and stimulating contribution which we might
perhaps sometime take the opportunity of debating:
  A matter of principle.
An interesting but wholly unrealistic concept, I'm afraid:
  A matter of high principle.
              In England now. *Lancet*, 20 October 1973

I used to imagine prospective speakers being catechised by
a BMA cliché committee to ensure they were properly
equipped for the rostrum.
  Q: What is immutable about principles?
  A: They are always basic.
  Q: Or alternatively?
  A: Fundamental.
  Q: Where does this moment invariably reside?
  A: In time.
  Q: In what manner must our messages be promulgated?
  A: They must go out.
  Q: Whence?
  Q: From this place.
  Q: In what manner?
  A: Loud.
  Q: And?
  A: Clear.
  Q: What is the only form of analysis we favour?
  A: The final.
  Q: And in that analysis what will happen to the truth?
  A: It will dawn.
  Q: At what inappropriate hour will that dawn take place?
  A: At the end of the day.
  Q: And what rustic omen will presage the event?
  A: The chickens will come home to roost.
  Anecdotal evidence. *Healthcare Management*, June 1994

Boots, size of

Measurement used by senior doctors to indicate a person's class
or status. Those who don't "know their place" or are uppity in

other ways, are said to be "too big for their boots". Phrase used almost exclusively by people who are too small for theirs.

Bottomley

Pejorative adjective applied to less savoury products of internal market.

The Right Hon Virginia Bottomley was Minister for Health (1989-92) and Secretary of State for Health (1992-5) when many of the NHS reforms bore fruit. She is remembered for her ill judged attempts to disguise what was happening with a mixture of soundbite, photo opportunity, and **echolalia**.

Bottomley ward
Hospital slang for corridors where patients are kept lying on trolleys when there are no beds.

Bottomley's children
Medical vernacular for:
1. "Psychiatric patients who sleep on pavements and in doorways throughout our land" (*BMA News Review*).
2. Young people, abandoned by family and state, who live in cardboard boxes in city centres.

Bowels, pride in control over

The archetypal English symptom. Few doctors have escaped the proud Englishman who, no matter how depressed he may seem during a consultation, will respond to the diffident inquiry "Bowels?" with a triumphant smile and a defiant: "Regular as clockwork, Doc".

> My wife has two topics of conversation: the Royal family and her bowels.
> Alan Bennett. *A Private Function* (screenplay), 1984

> My wife and I spent a holiday in a guest house. On our first evening when the guests assembled for dinner we were introduced to Auntie, 80 years old, a former nurse, neatly

dressed, and demure. The hostess announced that Auntie would say grace. All heads were reverently bowed and the silence broken by a clear authoritative voice: "O Lord. What we are about to receive, may it pass through us peacefully".

Dr Kerr Donald. *Personal communication*

Until the second world war, the English bowel culture was dominantly a middle class phenomenon, instilled in boarding schools whose inhabitants had to parade daily before the matron and answer the question "Been?"

But after the war, it spread rapidly through the lower orders, carried by returning soldiers who'd been brainwashed by officers like Apthorpe in Evelyn Waugh's *Men at Arms*, who never advanced nor retreated without his personal thunderbox.

The symptomatology of European chauvinism.
Rocket, Spring 1994

Although the situation is stressful, British citizens have been advised not to evacuate. The French have already evacuated and the Germans are threatening to do so.
World at One. Radio 4, June 1985.
(Correspondent in Teheran describing admirable example of British stoicism.)

Breakthrough

Dramatic breach of the frontiers of science reported in a medical journal.

Investigators at the Hospital del Salvador, Santiago, Chile, reported in the *BMJ* on August 30 that when 54 normal healthy people had one hand immersed in warm water the skin of 38 wrinkled and that of 16 did not. This, they vouchsafe, is "probably within the bounds of normal biological variation".
Bernard Dixon. Talking science.
World Medicine, 13 December 1980

Ability to lie on bed of nails not due to endogenous opioids.
Title of paper in *Lancet*, 24 May 1980. (The author acknowledged the help received from Esther Rantzen.)

Business plan

Tortuously written prospectus demanded from even the most unlikely departments in the new style NHS.

> Ted Cockayne, a GP in Bury St Edmunds has received a business prospectus from the West Suffolk Hospitals' Chaplaincy and Pastoral Care Department.
>
> It starts: "The department provides a comprehensive service which seeks to meet the spiritual/religious/pastoral needs of patients, relatives and staff within a framework of client choice appropriate to their cultural or religious expression (or none), and/or spiritual and pastoral need in accord with the first standard outlined in the Patient's Charter".
>
> And it concludes: "The department is committed to a developing quality strategy, departmental and clinical audit".
>
> Dr Cockayne asks: "How do you audit the chaplain?"
>
> I envisage a ceremony in which the chaplains are lined up on a suitable piece of West Suffolk greensward, the hospital chief executive prays for divine intervention, and then stands back to see which of his pastoral care providers is struck by a thunderbolt.
>
> Looking sideways. *Medical Monitor*, 6 November 1992

Care

(Obsolete) To show concern. To look after. What the NHS once used to do for the sick and infirm.

(Now) To allocate resources. Rarely used without qualifying adjective. As in:

Community care

A delusion. Belief in its existence seems directly related to the number of hours the deluded person has spent in the environs of Whitehall. A common political excuse for not providing care for the sick and the infirm.

Emergency care
The only form of care available in most hospitals in the second half of the financial year. A great nuisance to administrators.

Emergency admissions to hospitals have been rising. Such increases are disrupting the contractual system, distorting priorities by causing a shift in resources to pay for the increase, and making it difficult to plan for the future with confidence.
November newsletter published by the National Association of Health Authorities and Trusts 1994

Ongoing care
Tautologous phrase used in medical lectures, medical journals, hospital memoranda, and other places where the simple word is considered too lightweight. *See* BMAspeak, Trustspeak.

Social care
The care that doctors and hospitals gave to the sick and infirm before they grew obsessed with high technology. Demands high levels of personal skill from the carer. Hence:
Phrase used to excuse hospitals discharging the tediously sick and infirm to make room for those who will keep expensive capital equipment busy and in whom "outcome" is easier to measure. *See* Accountants.

Career structures

Shackles for the young designed by their elders. *See* Resentful Prisoner Syndrome.

Our academic masters, in their commendable desire to raise standards and to tidy things up, have laid too great a stress on neatness and behaved too often as if they were dealing with highly trained organisms and not with un-neat, quirky individuals.
The resentful prisoner game. *An Insider's Guide to the Games Doctors Play*, Gollancz, 1986

It's time we re-examined the concept that medicine is a lifetime commitment to one specialty rather than to a series

21

of tasks that serve the common purpose of our profession. Some people thrive on a lifetime commitment to one line of work. Others seem to commit themselves only because of anxiety about their professional identity. The challenge to postgraduate education is to promote enrichment at the expense of disenchantment.

One man's burden. *BMJ*, 22 January 1983

Rigid career structures are great promoters of mediocrity. I remember some years ago how a young surgical registrar, Peter Steele, took time off from medicine to join the Chris Bonnington expedition to Everest. When he returned, he applied for a job at a British hospital, and I've seen the letter he got in reply. In essence it asked why should the appointments committee, which had had many applications from people who had assiduously pursued an orthodox career, waste its time considering someone who had gone off and done something irrelevant like trying to climb Everest.

So Peter Steele went to Canada and British medicine, I believe, lost someone who had a lot to contribute to it.

The resentful prisoner game. *An Insider's Guide to the Games Doctors Play*, Gollancz, 1986

Caring professions

A self selected club. Membership most often claimed by doctors, nurses, and other one time patient treaters who have lost their enthusiasm for clinical medicine and sought refuge in medical politics and administration. Membership rarely claimed by those who actually look after patients.

Case conference

Official ceremony created in the late 1970s to maintain full employment in the **caring professions.**

Last week I attended a case conference to discuss whether a child should be taken into the care of the local authority. There were twenty persons present: one consultant, one senior medical officer, one general practitioner, one nursing officer, two health visitors, one legal adviser, one educational psychologist, one administrator from the education department, three school teachers, one educational welfare officer, one chief housing officer, one police sergeant, one divisional director of social services, two senior social workers, one social worker from the local authority, and one social worker from the child guidance clinic. Is this a record?

Harvey Marcovitch. *World Medicine*, April 1978

Casualty

Nostalgic programme transmitted by the BBC to remind people of services that were available at their local hospital before the department was closed.

Cause

Dangerous concept when dealing with disease. See **Illness**.

Lung cancer, as everyone knows, is most common among smokers...However, smokers who are unfortunate enough to inherit a gene for susceptibility are far more likely to contract cancer than are those who do not. If everybody smoked, lung cancer would be a genetic disease.

Steve Jones. *The Language of the Genes*, Flamingo, 1993

Cemetery

Underused educational facility.

My father, a GP in a Yorkshire colliery village, used to say that all doctors' houses should overlook cemeteries to remind them of their ultimate failure. When I was a medical student, he would say "Let's take a stroll amid my mistakes" and, while we walked, he would pass on ideas about medicine that have proved more enduringly practical than much I learned in medical school.

He would punctuate this tutorial by pausing in front of gravestones, sometimes to explain how the bones beneath might have lingered a little longer above the earth if he had been a little wiser, sometimes to illustrate the social

23

history of the village.

Mary T, aged 17, who died of septicaemia after an illegal abortion, lying alongside her father who suffocated underground in the big fire at Yorkshire Main the day before his daughter planned to tell him she was pregnant.

Ernie C, the colliery clerk who worked in the office and wore a stiff collar from Monday to Friday but on Saturday nights donned a black cloak and hood to wrestle in working men's clubs as The Rotherham Phantom.

Sometimes we paused on our walks just to adduce further evidence for my father's Law of Headstones: "The more unctuous the inscription, the more unscrupulous the rogue who lies beneath".

Body and soul. *Guardian*, July 1984

Chilblain

Odd blotch on skin rarely diagnosed outside England, maybe because the English like to see a manifestation of the dreaded chill.

The diagnosis is so out of fashion in other countries that when a group of Virginia doctors found red splotches on the thighs of plump young women who rode horses in the early morning cold—classic chilblains, according to Dr Renwick Vickers of Oxford—they thought they were describing a new disease, which they baptised "equestrian cold panniculitis".

Why are chilblains diagnosed so much more commonly in England than elsewhere? "The English think it is immoral to heat their houses much", said Dr Froom (a New York professor of family medicine).

Lynn Payer. *Medicine and Culture*, Gollancz, 1989

Child abuse

A genuine concern which dubious data turned into a witch hunt during the late 1980s and early '90s.

1986. Two Leeds paediatricians published an article entitled "Buggery in childhood". The test they used, "reflex anal dilatation", had not, at that time, been validated with

controls on normal children.
C J Hobbs, J M Wynne. Diagnosing sexual abuse, Lancet,
19 December 1987

1989. Two paediatricians from Birmingham reported that
the test was positive in 14% of small children. They
suggested that less than 1% of children are in fact
sodomised.
A Stanton, R Sunderland. Presence of reflux anal dilatation
in 200 children *BMJ*, 25 March 1989

[Using the Birmingham figures] the application of the reflex
anal dilatation test to 10 000 children would turn out 43 true
positives among 100 anally raped and 1386 false positives.
In other words, out of 100 "positive" tests, 97 would be false
positive. Words cannot describe the suffering of countless
families falsely accused of an unspeakable crime.
Petr Skrabanek. *The Death of Humane Medicine and the
Rise of Coercive Healthism*, The Social Affairs Unit, 1994

Satanic child abuse

Form of hysteria that erupted in Britain after the child abuse
epidemic. Accusations of abuse were pursued with enthusiasm;
denials by the accused and by the "victims" were construed as
admissions of guilt.

The worst excesses...have been perpetrated by social
workers determined to prove the existence of widespread
Satanic child abuse. Despite the lack of any police evidence
in support of these claims, the panic swept Britain. The
infiltration of social work by born again Christians and by
strong US fundamentalist influences has facilitated the
propaganda of a Satanic myth.
Petr Skrabanek. *The Death of Humane Medicine and the
Rise of Coercive Healthism*, The Social Affairs Unit, 1994

In 1991 a four year old girl and her brother developed skin
blisters after they had been shooting dried peas at each
other, with their father, through makeshift pea shooters
made from cow parsley stems. They were suffering from an
allergic reaction to cow parsley sap but the girl was
threatened with being taken into care. The family was not
believed and social workers ordered the girl to be kept in the
Royal London Trust Hospital for three days.
News report. *Independent*, 8 September 1991

A vigilant teacher in West Sussex noticed suspicious "bruises" on a six year old girl's legs and sent her to hospital where a paediatrician, a detective, and a social worker concluded that the "severe bruising" was inflicted either by a whip or a cane. The family was compelled to bring their other child to hospital for a humiliating examination for signs of "abuse". The child faced indefinite separation from her family until it was discovered she'd been wearing a new pair of wellingtons, with her name written in ink on the inside. The "bruises" washed off in the bath.

News report. *Times*, 22 February 1994

Cigarette

Source of only addictive lethal drug that can be sold legally on British streets. Successful peddlers are often honoured by Monarch or government.

Cigarette advertising

A good thing. Contributes to the nation's health by subsidising sport. Opposed only by European countries where, as all right thinking British politicians know, people don't know their ischial tuberosities from their olecranon processes.

Cigarette smoking

A bad thing. Commonest method of committing suicide. Kills over 100 000 Britons every year.

Clinical

Adjective used by football commentators to show that they can handle three syllable words.

The Oxford English Dictionary defines "clinical": "Latin clinicus, Greek κλῑνικός: of or pertaining to a bed".
So when football commentators say of a player, "Last

Saturday he produced a clinical finish", are we just being told that he scored in bed?

Medical Monitor, 20 March 1996

Clinical acumen

A form of wisdom that develops in doctors humble enough to learn from their mistakes. Those unprepared to learn dismiss it as lucky guesswork.

> Depend upon it, a lucky guess is never merely luck, there is always some talent in it.
> Jane Austen. *Emma*, 1816

Clinical errors

Mistakes some doctors are reluctant to admit, fearing that any confession of failure will subvert their claim to omniscience

> A fellow houseman, with me at the London Hospital, was clumsy with his hands but quick with his mind; he had a clever phrase for use after failing to put a needle into a patient's vein. "Now we do the other side", he used to remark in a satisfied voice; and the patients, if of moderately low mental calibre, would happily submit to what they believed was the other half of some bilateral investigation.
> Richard Asher. Medical salesmanship.
> *Middlesex Hospital Medical Journal*, February 1960

Clinical experience

Making the same mistakes with increasing confidence over an impressive number of years.

Coitus interruptus

Contraceptive technique that, when Englishmen talk to their doctors, becomes a rich source of regional euphemism and a confirmation of their abiding love of trains.

Cheshire and Merseyside—I get off the train at Edge Hill, doctor.

Cambridgeshire—I get out at Saffron Waldon.

Hampshire—I stop at Fratton.

Rural Sussex—I disembark at Haywards Heath.

London—I always change at Clapham Junction.

Colon

Lower bowel harbouring noxious substances that threaten the vitality of celebrities.

> Colonic irrigation seems to be regaining the social cachet it had in the 1930s. A recent *Sunday Times* article by Susan Clark, after hinting that Diana and Fergie were regular indulgers, continued:
>
> "Discretion is a key word among colonic therapists, who insist that client confidentiality precludes them from naming their patients but celebrity converts are said to include the author and yachtswoman Clare Francis, the actress Joan Collins, and Vidal Sassoon and his second wife, Ronnie".
>
> Odd, isn't it, how useful names always manage to breach the confidentiality barrier.
>
> *Medical Monitor*, 6 September 1995

> Blanche had two marketing ploys. The first was to imply that all the "best people "were her clients; the second was to let it be known that she was the county's only really high operator in a therapeutic field in which connoisseurs seem to measure efficacy in terms of altitude.
>
> The local GPs assumed that the arrival of the NHS would finish her off but instead it made her even richer because, with "specialists" and "operations" available to every Tom, Dick, and Harry, citizens of Higher Drive could maintain their social superiority only by indulging in treatments that were too expensive for the masses.
>
> Slagthorpe revisited. *World Medicine*, 23 February 1980

> You kindly wrote to me about this lady on 27.7.95 asking me to see her privately: I gathered from your letter that she had been using coffee for self administered colonic enemas.

She tells me that she feels better now and does not need to see me privately. Apparently the explanation is that her husband has bought her a new coffee percolator and she now feels better.

Medical Monitor, 20 September 1995

Colour coding

A way of simplifying administrative processes.

Some confusion has arisen about the new general ophthalmic services form. The white and pink copies should be sent to the GP together with the green copy. The white copy should be sent to the hospital with the green copy by the doctor. The pink copy should be kept on file by the GP. The yellow copy together with a photocopy of the green copy should be retained by the optician.
Torbay local medical committee newsletter.

Medical Monitor, 6 October 1993

Coloured water

1. Traditional quack remedy.
2. An alarming symptom.

A patient of mine in London on business thought he had cystitis. He went to a chemist who, unable to give him antibiotics, gave him some De Witts pills and advised him that they may discolour his urine. On his way back north, the man stopped at a service station and went to the gents where a small boy in the next stall stared wide eyed and unbelieving at the stream of bright blue urine.

"Hey, mister", he asked, "Why is your wee blue?"

With calm authority, the man replied: "I am not of this planet". Whereupon the boy rushed to the door shouting: "Dad, Dad, there's an alien in here".

Dr C M B Reid, Lytham GP.
Personal communication, 1996

Comedy

In the world inhabited by doctors, an inescapable ingredient of tragedy.

A GP friend used to look after an odd couple—a middle aged man and his elderly father—who lived together in an isolated house and who were as dependent on one another, and as argumentative, as Steptoe and son. One day the son called the doctor to see his father and when the GP went into the bedroom he found that the old man had died of a heart attack. He spent a minute or two trying to assemble the right words to break the news to the son who he knew loved his father more than he loved any creature on this earth. Yet when the doctor went downstairs he found, as so often happens, that he lapsed straight into platitude.

"I'm sorry to say", he muttered, "that your father has passed away".

"Bloody hell", said the son. "I've just made him a big plate of stew".

Heal thyself. Radio Four, August 1995

The most moving last words I know came from the playwright Brendan Behan, who died in a Dublin nursing home that was run by nuns. His final act on this earth was to look up at the young nun who sat by his bedside, clasp her by the hand, and whisper: "Thank you for being so kind to me. May you be the mother of a bishop".

Looking sideways. *Medical Monitor*, 29 September 1991

Committee

A group in which the politely diffident are manipulated by the politically ambitious.

A committee is a cul de sac down which ideas are lured and quietly strangled.

Sir Barnett Cocks. In: Winston Fletcher,
Meetings, meetings, Coronet, 1983

...a more advanced study [is] the differentiation of committee members into those whose self imposed mission is to govern (whether by divine or popular mandate) and those who truly seek the mystery of consensus.

In England now. *Lancet*, 20 October 1973

Overheard in a corridor in BMA House: "The speed with which this committee reacts is reminiscent of a hedgehog.

The big difference with a hedgehog is that all the pricks are on the outside".

Medical Monitor, 8 February 1995

Committee consensus

Compromise achieved when the politely diffident accept that the only way they'll get out of the room is to endorse the views of the politically ambitious.

Committee games

Diversions which the politely diffident use to insulate themselves from the mind numbing proceedings.

Inventaproverb
A game for two or more players devised by Jeremy Bullmore when chairman of J Walter Thompson.

> Before the meeting each player has to create a saying that sounds wise and aphoristic but is in truth meaningless. They then have to drag it sententiously into the discussion, scoring a point only if the non-players accept it as relevant or even thoughtful. Bullmore's original creation was "Somebody has to bury the undertaker". Others include "It may not be the man who saws the logs who needs the fire" and "Success is merely failure in reverse", which you can, of course, also use the other way round. The secret of success is to get the tone of voice right.
> One man's burden. *BMJ*, 16 February 1985

Interrogative blocking
This can halt even the most intransigent of bores. The question should sound relevant while being unanswerable.

> Yes, but that isn't really what we're discussing, is it?
> Stephen Potter. *Lifemanship*, Hart-Davis, 1947

The transferred question
This incites arguments between others and allows you to sit back and enjoy the squabble you've created.

> "Personally I don't feel strongly about this but I don't

31

understand how you can ignore what Professor Catchall just said".

"Surely what Charles is saying, chairman, is that your report ducks the issue".

Anecdotal evidence.
Healthcare Management, November 1993

Statements camouflaged as questions

These can be used to introduce uncertain—or, even better, invented—data:

"Surely it was established some time ago that the normal is 19.79?"

"Isn't he the chap who caused all the trouble at Manchester?"

And if anyone questions the data you've introduced, you come back immediately with the second part of the "Double Whammy".

"Do you mean you just don't care about these figures?"

"Aren't you at all interested in what happens to the patients?"

"Doesn't it worry you that the theatres are unsafe?"

Ibid

Committeespiel

The blend of language and intonation that committee persons know will carry them to the top. The art of making the right sort of noise ... literally.

Experienced committeespielers know that, if they keep rhubarbing away in the right sort of monotone, their audience will soon become hypnotised by the sound of the words and lose grasp of their meaning.

I once heard a GMC president, John Walton, finish off a protracted monologue with the sentence: "Of course, I'm just talking out loud". And, because the words made the right sort of noise, those who sat round the table nodded in agreement as if they were in the presence of profundity.

Anecdotal evidence. *Healthcare Management*, October 1994

In this malignant hypertrophy of language nobody says anything, they "state", or worse still they "intimate that". They never think, they "are of the opinion that"; nobody finishes anything, it is "duly completed"; nobody ever looks ahead, they "envisage a long term policy". This language is a waste of duplicating paper and a waste of time. Incompetence can hide behind its opacity and activity be smothered by its voluminous folds. May I warn you of this deadly and contagious miasma. May I personally intimate to you that after due consideration I am of the opinion that it should be an integral part of your basic policy to take due precautionary measures against the obnoxious prolixity. Richard Asher.

Richard Asher Talking Sense, Pitman Medical, 1972

Communication, breakdown in

Commonest excuse for catastrophic balls-ups that could be more accurately described as "a breakdown in understanding" or "sheer bloody incompetence".

Because communicating is something that people do and not a personal attribute the phrase protects the guilty from accusations of personal failing.

Large commercial enterprises, and even political parties, who find that people mistrust them, or dislike what they say, are slow to admit that may have made wrong judgments. They prefer to think that their "message" is not "getting across". In order to be loved, they tell themselves, all they need to do is "communicate". They may well be right but, sadly, when they call in the communications "experts" too often all they learn is a bunch of public relations tricks, which are fun to use but generate little understanding.

One man's burden. *BMJ*, 22 March 1986

Communication skills

1. Chic subject to include in an undergraduate postgraduate curriculum. These days there are so many courses in

"communication" you need to be very lucky to escape one.

For some 30 years, I've worked with people who earn their living as what others call "communicators". Those who do it rarely use the title and I suspect the aggrandising of the simple process of getting people to understand what you mean has itself become a barrier. Calling it "communication" suggests there is something difficult about it—complicated techniques to be learned, a new academic discipline to be mastered—when all most people need to do is develop personal qualities they already have and gain the confidence to use them...

The quality we should be striving for is not communication but understanding.

One man's burden. *BMJ*, 22 March 1986

2. Skills that teachers are better at advocating than using.

Tim Albert, a journalist who runs courses for doctors and administrators who want to write more clearly, quotes a sentence used by a London medical school to advertise its course in communication skills:

"In order to maximise learning opportunities participants should, in their own interests, bring one or two pieces of work for the course tutor to enable him to structure the course accordingly".

Albert wonders why they didn't write: "If you want to get the most out of the course, bring some examples of your work".

Anecdotal evidence.
Healthcare Management, December 1994

The most valuable qualities are a sensitivity to the emotions and reactions of others and an awareness of the way that what we say and do appears to them. The understanding needed to develop those qualities is, I submit, more likely to be absorbed from novels, films, and plays than from textbooks on communication skills.

One advantage of novels is that they are likely to be better written and easier to read than textbooks, and one of my happiest memories of the communications business is of four students sleeping soundly in a lecture theatre while their teacher of "communication skills" trundled his lecture along its predetermined groove.

One man's burden. *BMJ*, 22 March 1986

Community

Subversive philosophical notion that distorts right thinking about health care.

First Mrs Thatcher declared there was no such thing as society. Now, we were told at a meeting of psychiatrists last month, Mr Dorrell has instructed officials at the Department of Health not to use the word "community" because it has developed "negative connotations".

The news led to much speculation at the meeting about what should happen to academics lumbered with politically incorrect titles like Professor of Community Psychiatry.

One suggestion was that they should go for the portmanteau option and become Professors of Neglected Schizophrenics, Non-BUPA-Subscribing Cardboard Box Dwellers, and Other NHS Rejects Psychiatry.

Medical Monitor, 16 October 1996

Compensation

Arrangement by which lawyers get doctors to pay for lawyers' mistakes.

When Thomas Passmore of Norfolk, Virginia, thought his right hand was possessed by the devil, he cut it off with a circular saw. He had seen the malignant number 666 appear on it so he followed the biblical injunction: "If thine right hand offend thee, cut it off". When he, and his hand, were taken to a local hospital, he refused permission for the surgeons to intervene because the bible offered no authority for the surgical reattachment of offending body parts.

The hospital sought to override his instructions with a court injunction on the grounds that he was grossly deluded and incapable of making a rational decision.

The judge refused to grant an injunction. Mr Passmore is now suing the hospital for $3.4 million for obeying his instructions.

Anecdotal evidence. *Medical Interface*, September 1996

Complementary medicine

Play therapy for doctors worn down by the demands of the scientific method. Sometimes confused with **alternative medi-**

35

cine, which is similar to complementary medicine but more profitable. *See also* Holistic medicine, More holistic than thou.

> The same rigorous study should apply to both orthodox and complementary medicine, so why the need for the division? If a therapy is found to be effective it is automatically a part of medicine. If a suggested therapy is found to be ineffective, it is not medicine. There is no advantage, and much disadvantage, for progress in the art and science of medicine in maintaining such a meaningless division.
> R Edgar Hope-Simpson. Letter, *British Journal of General Practice*, December 1995

Compliance

Commendable obedience in patients. Harks back to days when doctors issued Doctor's Orders, which patients were expected to obey.

> Patients who take their medicine like a man are described as "showing a high level of compliance". Those who reject their doctor's treatment or advice suffer from "non-compliance"—clearly a failure on the part of the patient, not of the doctor.
> One man's burden. *BMJ*, 28 January 1984

Linked to two other words that doctors take in their unthinking stride:

Consent
Implies that patients have been given a choice when all they have been offered is the chance to acquiesce to someone else's choice.

Cooperative
Sensible attitude of patients who unquestioningly follow their doctor's advice.

The trio is linked by definition: a cooperative patient is one who first consents and then complies.

Computer error

Useful scapegoat for administrative cock ups. Computers, like other deities, cannot be fined, admonished, or forced to resign.

Board Policy. A cornerstone of Horton Trust policy, it seems, is that notice boards should "reflect a professional approach in keeping with the Corporate image". And boards "must meet with the maintenance guidelines issued by the literature work group".

The joy of finding a bureaucracy setting literary standards quickly faded when a subsequent sentence, ungrammatical and oddly punctuated, revealed what the "literature work-group" was really up to. "All in-house notices must comply with the literature guidelines, in order that the corporate image is maintained".

Anecdotal evidence.
Healthcare Management, February 1994

Corporate tyranny

Top people's version of mob rule. Phrase coined by Sir Douglas Black to describe how when people band together they are capable of follies that, as individuals, they would not perpetrate on other individuals.

Relative precepts are treated as absolute commandments, the "public interest" is preferred to individual welfare, and no distinction is made between different degrees of misdemeanour.

Douglas Black. Widow is a victim of "corporate tyranny".
Letter, *BMJ*, 11 January 1997

I see an example of this in the recent refusal to allow a widow to use semen taken from her husband during his final illness in an attempt to have the child that they both wanted. The Human Fertilisation and Embryological Authority is of course legally correct and has the comfort of a High Court assurance to that effect...(but) it seems to me that this is a case in which the distress and hardship to an individual are glaringly obvious and the value to society, still less to any one person, minimal.

Ibid

Cosmetic surgeons

Plastic surgeons who trained to do good, then learned to do well.

In the US, physical image is now more important than

mental cleanliness, and cosmetic surgeons have taken over from psychiatrists as purveyors of the American Dream. Success is no longer a matter of letting it all hang out but of having it all tucked in.

Every day, it seems, more Americans realise it is not inhibitions that are holding them back but baggy eyelids, baldness, or sagging boobs.

At meetings of American cosmetic surgeons, the high seriousness of the scientific programme is invariably enhanced by the whispered observations exchanged in the hotel lobbies. "Guess whose nose he just got...There goes the boob king of San Diego...That guy's reslung half the asses in Beverly Hills".

If the face doesn't fit. *Medical Punch*, March 1983

I was once handed visiting cards by a couple of plastic surgeons in Los Angeles. The back of one card carried a cartoon of an ape faced man saying: "Don't envy a good complexion, buy one", and on the back of the other was a cartoon of a woman sitting *en neglige* in front of her dressing table and saying: "Mirror, mirror on the wall...lie to me".

Audiomonitor, March 1995

Few people in Southern California have inhibitions about their cosmetic operations. Dammit all, the surgery is so expensive you want folks to know you can afford it. A woman who has had a face job, a nose job, a chin job, or a boob job will give a cocktail party for her plastic surgeon just as soon as the scars have healed and invite her friends round so she can show off what he's done for her.

The surgeons, whose role hovers uneasily twixt that of doctor and gigolo, are delighted to attend because these show off parties are where they recruit most of their future customers...a sort of surgical Tupperware technique.

The American dream. *An Insider's Guide to the Games Doctors Play*, Gollancz, 1986

Coudé catheter

Urinary catheter with a *coud* (bend) in it. Traditionally used for the drawing of water and the teasing of medical students. The second usage was apparently unknown to one of the 20th century's most prolific authors of surgical textbooks, Hamilton

Bailey. His reaction when the students teased back provoked a letter of memorable pomposity.

> Sir,—In volume 6 of the winter number of *The Leech*—the journal of the Cardiff Medical Students' Club—there appeared an article on Emile Coudé, 1800-70, a surgeon of Niort, France, who, it was alleged, invented, and in 1835 published an account of, the coudé catheter. This biography was written in a serious and restrained vein, and was replete with two references, one to the autobiography of Emile Coudé, and another to *Le Mois Medical* for a description of the invention. In addition, the article contained a reproduction of a woodcut purporting to be a likeness of the inventor.
>
> We have been able to prove that the whole of this article is a fabrication and the references are fictitious. To expose this deception is of practical importance. As a result of the hoax, a number of pages of the 11th edition of *A Short Practice of Surgery* that were passed for press have had to be reset in as far as the capital "C" of Coudé is concerned, and biographical footnotes to Emile Coudé deleted.
>
> To save others from falling into this mire, we hope that you will publish this letter.
>
> Clifford Morson, president, Socit Internationale; Hamilton Bailey; W J Bishop, editor, Medical History, A d'Urologie.
>
> *BMJ*, 23 August 1958

Counselling

Fashionable but ill defined therapy for those suffering from a condition for which medicine can't offer a quick fix. Doctors at their wits' end trying to cope with a patient's problems can recommend "counselling" and feel they've done something. *See* Management.

> Reviewing my clinical notes, I discovered how my patients interpreted three words I'd got into the habit of using.
> Advised: The doctor told me what to do.
> Discussed: I didn't fancy what the doctor recommended, but she persuaded me.
> Counselled: The doctor didn't seem to know what to do.
> Judith Harvey. *Healthcare Management*, April 1994

I gave up visiting my psychoanalyst because he was

meddling too much in my private life.

Tennessee Williams.
Quoted in Medical Monitor, 19 February 1997

Not be confused with **sympathetic listening** (now obsolete). In less enlightened times kindly persons tried to help victims of stress or tragedy by listening to their troubles, giving them useful information, or even, whisper it gently, just by talking to them.

> Ever since communication became an industry—ever since communication became communications, and conversation dwindled into something people listed as an interest, along with stamp collecting or keeping ferrets—above all, since the spoken word was taken into public ownership by the media and began to fill the universe with a sort of roaring— ever since that time, confidence that there is an individual to talk to has waned in exact proportion to confidence that it is an individual who is talking.
> . . . I suspect each of us from time to time feels marooned in the electronic nowhere, and at such moments we may find ourselves thinking with a mixture of wistfulness and hope of a day when men actually turned to each other as Johnson first turned to Boswell, and in an exchange of words that celebrated and embraced the possibility of their joint existences, cried, "Give me your hand. I have taken a liking to you."
>
> Robert Robinson.
> *A presidential address to the Johnson Society of Lichfield,*
> 1982

Professional counsellor
Self awarded title assumed by busybodies who turn up at scenes of national tragedy eager to inflict unasked for advice on people whose real need is for sympathetic contact with normal human beings.

Creative dysphasia

Common speech disorder. A form of **Malaproposis** in which the surrogate word actually enhances the meaning. First described by Simon Dean, a GP in Bury St Edmunds, after a woman had said to him: "I think I have thrush doctor. Could I have one of those clandestine pessaries?"

I think my husband's got Old Timer's Disease.
Audiomonitor, November 1995

One of Ian Soutar's Edinburgh patients described himself as suffering from "carnal tunnel syndrome". Dr Soutar treated him, naturally, with a cock-up splint.
Medical Monitor, 2 October 1976

A woman came to see me this week with a lump on her head. She said she came from a "lumpy family" and her mother had suffered from herbaceous cysts. My partner, Elizabeth Meinhard, had seen her last year with a similar lump and wondered, when she returned, if this were a perennial problem.
Richard Lynch-Blosse, Abingdon. *Personal communication*

Dr Jim McCracken of Nottingham has heard attenders at the antenatal clinic ask for repeat prescriptions of their "frolic acid tablets" or their equally titillating "phallic acid tablets".
Medical Monitor, 8 January 1993

A patient in Small Heath, Birmingham, who was vomiting blood and had a long history of heavy alcohol consumption, explained to Dr R G Harrison that he'd been diagnosed as having a "ferocious liver".

Another, who had pain on defecation, wanted a repeat prescription of cream for her "fisherman's halo".
Medical Monitor, 6 March 1996

A teenage girl had been brought by her mother to Rachel Gatrill's surgery at Wells in Somerset, because she was suffering from cyclical pelvic pain. At a crucial moment in the consultation, the mother leaned towards the doctor and whispered: "We've already been told that she has Messerchmidts but this seems to be something else".

For a moment, says Dr Gatrill, she wondered if it might be Hurricanes or Spitfires.
Audiomonitor, November 1995

Creative dysgraphia
Dysfunction similar to creative dysphasia but affecting writing.

From Cheltenham, Dr I M L Terrell sends the first report of a terrifying new zoonosis. A patient arriving for an insurance examination had recorded in his past medical history: "Operation to remove voracious seal from left scrotum".

Medical Monitor, 1 May 1996

Mark Davis of Sidcup received this specialist report on a patient with persistent hyperacidity: "His reflux symptoms were kept under control with antisecretary therapy"—an antidyspeptic measure that I suspect is underused.

Medical Monitor, 2 October 1996

I gather that she does have a habit of lying on the grass, which may predispose her to incest bites.

Letter from a psychiatrist
to Dr Stephen John Forsdick of St Austell

Bhasker Patel of Hounslow found this on a claim form:
What is your illness or disability?
A: Sealine diamenton.
Say no more, squire.

Medical Monitor, 13 November 1996

Crocodile concern

(After crocodile tears.) Solemn air assumed by nostrum pedlars.

"I've got to have an operation," says an overworried man.
Below him comes an explanatory broken sentence:
More serious than most men realise...
...the troubles caused by harsh toilet tissue.

Life Magazine. Advertisement, 1941

Drawing of a man who is clearly a social outcast: haggard, shame faced, and unable to look the artist in the eye. The line below spells out his crime.
He took his girl to the swimming bath and gave her ATHLETE'S FOOT.
He was...A CARRIER.

Life magazine. Advertisement, 1943

I dearly love a non sequitur if it's operatic enough, and, marooned overnight in the city of Washington, I turned on the television and caught the opening lines of one of the commercials. The scene was a bus stop and it was raining,

and the man standing there with his umbrella turned to the
camera and said, "In weather like this, diarrhoea's no fun".
For sheer quality, no programme was going to match that, so
I turned it off and went to bed.

Robert Robinson. *The Dog Chairman*, Allen Lane, 1982

Cruciate position

Alignment that occurs when the patient is horizontal and the
doctor vertical. Professor Neil Kessel, who coined the term,
points out that no useful communication can occur in this
position.

Modified Cruciate Position

Gynaecologist's version of the traditional cruciate. The patient
remains horizontal but the doctor sits with attention focused on
places other than the patient's face.

> A distinguished English actress had her first baby in a
> teaching hospital that prides itself on its teaching of
> communication skills. She'd had an episiotomy so her legs
> were raised into the stirrups when the houseman arrived to
> repair her perineum. He acknowledged her presence with a
> gruff "Good morning" then settled on his stool and stitched
> away, his attention, in her words, "wholly fixed on his site
> of action".
>
> After several minutes of silent stitching, and no doubt
> feeling the need to exercise his communication skills, he
> asked without raising his head: "Haven't I seen you on
> television?"
>
> Anecdotal evidence.
> *Healthcare Management*, October 1994

Decent chap

Accolade that senior doctors bestow on juniors (of both sexes) of
whom they approve. *See* Sound.

A good move is to get a job at one of those hospitals that call themselves "centres of excellence". Before you apply, find out what sort of person they're after: a "brain", a scrum half, a freemason, or even the statutory black or woman they're prepared to engage in these permissive times. Most likely they will be after a decent chap known to one of the consultants or recommended to him by another decent chap at another decent place. That's the job to go for, using all the arse-crawling ploys you picked up at medical school.

Body and soul. *Guardian*, February 1986

Decent thing, being seen to do the

Acting in a way that will impress senior doctors who can offer you patronage and preferment. *See* Sound.

The son of George Bernard Shaw's chiropractor—how's that for a tenuous connection?—once showed me this paragraph from a letter the old boy had sent to the *Times*.

"English decency is a rather dirty thing. It is responsible for more indecency than anything else in the world. It is a string of taboos. You must not mention this; you must not appear conscious of that; you must not meddle with the other—at least, not in public. And the consequence is that everything that must not be mentioned in public is mentioned in private as a naughty joke".

The *Times* did the decent thing and refused to publish it.

Medical Monitor, May 1997

Decorated Municipal Gothic

A prose style that evolves when writers eschew simple words that might express their ideas in a neat and palatable form and use instead language they believe adds dignity, scientific worth, or even grandeur to their utterance.

This vehicle is being utilised for highway cleansing purposes.
Notice on back of municipal dustcart in Cheltenham, 1967

The tendency to dress up ideas in long rumbling words of high prestige value is illustrated by this quotation:

"The pragmatic verity of the physiological concept of

disease is established by its usefulness: with functional integrity our goal the no-thoroughfare of unattainable structural integrity leaves us no longer at a therapeutic nonplus".

C Mawdsley. Medical pudder. *Res Medica*, Summer 1968

In a recent paper the author wants to tell us that his patient was fed, but writes: "alimentation was maintained".

Ibid

Four months ago a doctor wrote an article about bed wetting in which he drew a distinction between better educated people who plan a small but successful family and those with lower standards who raise large mediocre families. This is the way he put it (but I have condensed it a good deal).

"The mobile families described as showing a loose-knit kinship network and shared conjugal roles accept occupational emancipation and its consequences on interpersonal relationships. They determine the number of their children by a critical assessment of their own emotional, social and economic potential, and they strive to create one or two competitively successful children rather than a gregarious egalitarian sibling group".

Well I ask you? When you take your family on holiday, do you say "I am taking my gregarious egalitarian sibling group with me?" Did some of you play an excellent card game in your childhood called Happy Families? Do you think you would have enjoyed it more if it was called Euphoric Gregarious Egalitarian Sibling Groups?

Richard Asher. *Richard Asher Talking Sense*,
Pitman Medical, 1972

The indefatigable Tim Albert, who started by teaching doctors how to write clearly and is now employed by medical institutions to bring meaning to their utterances, came across this piece of NHS "communication".

"The whole purpose of reaching agreement in respect of maintaining disagreements that occur within an internal framework has been known for many years. We would therefore ask you on this occasion as we have done in the past to continue to use the further stages in the internal procedure if you so desire in order that no accusations can be levelled at either side for failing to abide by agreements."

"Does it mean", asks the impertinent Albert, "Please

follow the internal grievance procedure?"

Medical Monitor, 20 September 1995

Nagging away in the back of one's mind there is always the suspicion that these people may really have nothing to say, and that mere words are all they have to offer, that the medium is in fact the message. It is a matter of experience and observation that someone with a genuine piece of information can usually manage to communicate it in a reasonably straightforward and intelligible way. The verbal nonsense tends to come from people with nothing to say, but with a powerful vested interest in saying it impressively.

Kenneth Hudson.
The Dictionary of Diseased English, Papermac, 1977

Dedication

The deep devotion doctors show at the front of books that they write.

Most dedications are sentimental:

To my mother...and my father...who helped me to become a physician and who always encouraged me in the pursuit of knowledge.

Mircea Morariu. *Major Neurological Syndromes*,
Charles C Publishers,1979

To the martyrs of medicine—the physician's family.

Shahbudin Rahimtoola.
Infective Endocarditis, Grune and Stratton,1978

We dedicate this book to each other since, against all odds, we remained friends during its production.

James Mead, Armand Fulco. *The Unsaturated and Polyunsaturated Fatty Acids in Health and Disease*,
Charles C Publishers, 1976

Some are chauvinistic:

To...our wives, who do not know the convex from the concave side of a contact lens, but were good enough sports to keep us supplied with free time and coffee while we were working on this book.

Harold Stein, Bernard Slatt. *Fitting Guide for Hard and Soft Contact Lenses: a Practical Approach*, Mosby C V, 1977

Others are powerfully scented with midnight oil:

> Homage is herewith paid
> To those hordes who still seek aid
> For lingering dissatisfactions
> With lenses, frames, or their refractions.
> Benjamin Milder. *The Fine Art of Prescribing Glasses*
> *without Making a Spectacle of Yourself*, Triad, 1978

And a few are imaginative:

To my family

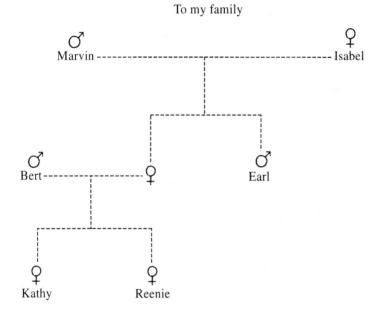

Lucille Whaley. *Understanding Inherited Disorders*,
Mosby C V, 1974

Deferred

Not done and unlikely to be done.

Degrees

Letters that eccentric non-American universities encourage doctors to put after their names to confuse information technologists.

A heavily "personalised" letter from BMA Services selling its Discount Connection, and addressed to Mr J C M Strachan FRCS Ed, began "Dear Mr Ed".

Medical Monitor, 28 May 1997

A paper in the *Lancet* by E Farquhar Buzzard, MB Oxon, is referenced in the *Cumulative Index Medicus* as a joint publication by Buzzard EF and Oxon MB. The index also includes MB's elder brother, DM Oxon, and his cousins, MB Lond and ChB Cantab. (The emphatic use of the middle initial suggests that Charles B has emigrated to the US.)

Even more oddly, the authors of a paper on gastric ulceration are given as DuPlessis DJ and W'srand CM.

Looking sideways. *Medical Monitor*, 28 September 1990

One of the targets for a computerised recruiting drive by the New York Academy of Sciences was Stuart Carne, former president of the Royal College of General Practitioners. The recruiting letter included a replica, "greatly reduced", of the Certificate, "suitable for framing", he would receive when he paid up.

The name on the certificate inscribed in Gothic Script "in recognition of and certification of being elected" was: "Stuart Frcgp".

He wrote asking for help with the pronunciation of his surname.

Medical Monitor, 19 February 1997

You have to feel sympathy for the group that published a paper entitled: *Cardiac action of vasoactive polypeptides in the rat. I. Bradykinin. II. Angiotensin.* For months their department was flooded with reprint requests addressed to Dr I Bradykinin.

Looking sideways. *Medical Monitor*, 28 September 1990

de Vries Effect

Natural decline in the rate of marital coition. *See* Beans-in-a-jar hypothesis. Name devised by Dr William H James after reading a paragraph in a de Vries novel.

> Sex in marriage is like a medicine. Three times a day for the first week. Then once a day for another week. Then once every three or four days until the condition has cleared up.
>
> Peter de Vries. *Witch's Milk*, Gollancz, 1975

Dignitary

Caption writer's label for a worthy about whom there is nothing else to say. Has nothing in common with dignity save five consonants and two vowels. Crops up in local newspapers during BMA annual meetings.

> Anyone who has seen a clutch of our self important colleagues tripping over their gold chains, or sweating it out under their ermine in the noonday sun, knows that the medical dignitary can be an even more ludicrous animal than the civic variety. Some quirk of medical anatomy makes academic finery sit uneasily upon our person. Lawyers can just get away with it because they wear wigs. Maybe doctors should follow their example, for whenever I see that collection of best suits and multicoloured robes that assembles for Grand Medical Occasions, I'm reminded of the chorus of the Slagthorpe and District Operatic and Thespian Society standing by to give us an earful of Rudolf Friml.
>
> Anecdotal evidence. *Medical Interface*, February 1996

> There is a natural law that the lesser the honour the greater the pride in its possession. Dean Acheson, the American statesman, was intercepted in the lobby of a Washington hotel by a flustered lady who had jammed the zip in her ball gown.
>
> Acheson managed to unstick it and, after thanking him, the lady said: "I think I should tell you I am a regional assistant state vice president of the Daughters of the American Revolution".
>
> Said Acheson: "My dear lady what a moment ago was a rare privilege now appears to have been a great honour".
>
> Looking sideways. *Medical Monitor*, 2 November 1990

Dirty docs

Jack the Lads who appear before the GMC to provide entertainment for newspaper readers. *See* Blonde.

> When MRC sociologists studied newspaper coverage of GMC disciplinary procedures they found that male doctors were portrayed as professional men succumbing to their

natural urges while the image of the other woman was of someone who had betrayed her partner and family.

"This jokey, nudge-nudge-wink-wink attitude to the hearings is also demonstrated in the cartoons. Of the four cartoons in our sample three show very busty young women, two without clothes, submitting to their doctor's attentions".

Favourite headlines on the cases included Dirty Doc, Doctor Grope, Romeo Doc, Carry On Doc, and Fruity Doc.

Medical Monitor, 5 March 1997

Disorientated

More confused than the doctor.

Doctor's note

The ultimate verification.

> We have been instructed to act in the administration of the estate of the above named deceased. Following Mr X's death the Executors now wish to cancel a holiday booking which Mr and Mrs X had made in September of this year and which was to be taken during the Christmas holiday. We completed the insurance claim form and had forwarded this to the insurance company together with the original Death Certificate.
>
> The insurance company have, however, advised that the Death Certificate is insufficient for their purposes and have requested that the Medical Certificate on the reverse side of the insurance claim form be completed by Mr X's usual doctor.
>
> *Solicitor's letter to Dr J M Griffin,*
> *a Northampton GP, 1995*

Domestic pets

Sometimes regarded as surrogate children. Now recognised as surrogate spouses

> When asked why she never married, the novelist Marie

Corelli was said to have replied that she had three pets who took the place of a man: a dog that growled all morning, a parrot that swore all evening and a cat that stayed out all night.

Celia Ennis. Letter, *Times*, 5 February 1997

Double negative

Stylistic device favoured by medical authors in need of assertiveness training. *See* Negativism

> There are consultants of a certain age who think a double negative adds dignity to their prose. "The diagnosis is probably a peptic ulcer but neoplasm is a not unlikely possibility".
>
> They suffer from what George Orwell described as the Not-un Syndrome. He offered the definitive sentence: "A not unblack dog chased a not unsmall rabbit across a not ungreen field".
>
> *Medical Monitor*, 20 March 1996

> Browsing through the *BMJ* (2 April 1994) Dougal Jeffries, who practices in Salisbury, stumbled upon a rare syntactical specimen—not just a double but a quadruple negative.
>
> "Having thrown out the motion to rescind last year's decision to stop opposing fundholding, the conference..."
>
> It's a particularly fine example, says Dr Jeffries, because it contains no "not"s, just four negative transitive verbs.
>
> *Monitor Weekly*, 14 September 1994

Echolalia

The politician's way of dealing with the NHS. Defined in the OED: "The meaningless repetition of words and phrases".

> The hospital I visited as a child was a place of order and discipline and hygiene and reassurance. The hospital I visited this week was a place of grime and suppressed chaos.

55

"Ah, but London hospitals have special problems..." (said Mrs Bottomley) .

"I had to wait three weeks for an *x* ray result..."

"We are doing five hips for every four done three years ago..."(said Mrs Bottomley).

We are in two worlds, she in that sunlit upland of rising graphs and improving figures, we in that zone of queues and cancellations, postponed operations, and trolleys in corridors.

> Martyn Harris. Interview with Virginia Bottomley,
> *Daily Telegraph*, 30 January 1995

Education

Elitist activity. Cost ineffective. Unpopular with **Grey Suits**. Now largely replaced by **training**.

> To be trained is to have arrived; to be educated is to continue to travel...a challenge to get better all the time.
> Kenneth Calman. *Utopia and Other Destinations*,
> BBC Radio 4, 29 March 1997

Educationalist

Title assumed by teachers who seek to come to terms with their own failure by formulating rules for others and evolving a language all their own.

> "Either he met the students during crisis intervention sessions", Susan said to me on the telephone, "Or at coordinative evaluation conferences or he's been a resource person during attempts at therapeutic redirection".
>
> "You are, I hope, quoting", I said.
>
> "You mean the jargon? You hear it so much you get used to it".
>
> "Talking like that will rot your teeth", I said.
> Robert B Parker. *Ceremony*, Penguin, 1982

> Letter from applicant wanting to teach 10 year old children:
>
> I enjoy the dynamism of the contemporary education scene and consider the logistical and political frustrations

that inevitably occur as a constant cognitive challenge. My teaching is well prepared and planned, with an emphasis upon flexibility within a structure. Through this, I aim to develop relationships which will nurture the child beyond legal criteria, exploring both the academic potential and aesthetic dimensions of human engagement. Also, in studying a wide range of philosophies in education, I am refining an ability to think dialectically, absorbing the pertinence of new ideas, and allowing them to permeate through tried and tested good practice where appropriate. To this end, I have recently been labelled by my tutor as an "eclectic progressive".

Monitor Weekly, 8 June 1994

Empathy

Human quality best deployed by those who haven't been on a course in it.

Letter from psychiatric social worker to parents of child attending an Oxfordshire child guidance clinic:
I would be happy to offer you an appointment at 3pm on the 15th of next month in order that we may work out together a task centred goal orientated approach which will hopefully build up X's strength and self-confidence. Hope to see you then. Go well. Yours sincerely,
Anecdotal evidence. *Healthcare Management*, March 1994

Empowerment

Word used to persuade the politically correct that you are involving others in decisions while actually making them yourself.

End of day

Moment in time often invoked in medicopolitical rhetoric.

A retired surgeon, Horace Fleming of Enniskillen, once suggested that the best way to discomfit users of rhetorical clichés was to repeat the sentiment using different words. Thus "at the end of the day" became "at the beginning of the night".

One man's burden. *BMJ*, 29 September 1984

Epigraph

Opportunity to pass a meaningful message to those you leave behind.

My father was a GP in Yorkshire and I still feel guilty that, after his death, we didn't fulfil a wish he'd expressed one evening after he'd had a good dinner with a couple of doctor friends.

Egged on by them, he'd described the headstone he would like to see erected over his grave. It was to be a simple slab of Connemara marble with an electric bell embedded in its centre. And beneath the bell-push would be the carved inscription:

You can ring like hell but you can't get me now.

Yours in peace.

James Michael O'Donnell

Anecdotal evidence. *Healthcare Management*, June 1994

Eponym

Easiest way for doctors to achieve immortality. *See* Scruffie's Triangle.

I feel like the man in a Thurber cartoon who rushes into a doctor's surgery shouting "I've got Bright's disease and he's got mine".

Milton Shulman. *Stop the Week*.

BBC Radio 4, December 1991

GPs are ideally placed to achieve fame through eponymity because they see vast numbers of patients with indeterminate symptoms. All you need to do is make a collection of a few of those symptoms, label it as a syndrome, and then attach your name. But show discretion in your choice of symptoms. You don't want to suffer the eponymous fate of Thomas Crapper.

Anecdotal evidence. *Medical Interface*, March 1996

If you don't mind sharing immortality, why not share an eponym with a chum? The more names that are attached to a syndrome, the more impressive it becomes. Ideally you should choose a chum with a complicated name. This will add intellectual weight. Conditions with names that are difficult to pronounce are thought to present conceptual difficulties. Creutzfeld-Jakob disease, for instance, acquires gravitas from its label.

Once again, however, you need to show discretion. Don't go over the top as in "the Finsterer-Lake-Lahey modification of the Miculicz-Kronlein-Hofmeister-Reichal-Polya improvement of the Billroth II gastrectomy".

Ibid

Dr R Grant describes (*Scot Med J* 1987;32:57-9) the neurological assault on the big toe that began when French and German neurologists staked rival claims to one of neurology's enduring signs—the extensor plantar response. When Joseph Francois Felix Babinski described his discovery in 1896, no one thought it important but, within a few years, enthusiasm for scratching, pinching, and stroking the foot was pandemic in Europe.

The heavyweight pretenders to Babinski's title were two German neurologists, Professors Oppenheim and Schaefer, who refused to accept that their eponymous reflexes were mere modifications of the Babinski original.

In the early 1900s, Americans began to "discover" different ways of eliciting the response, and eponymous claims for inducing movement of the big toe now include Bing's sign (pricking the dorsum of the foot), Strumpell's phenomenon (resulting from pressure over the anterior tibia), Cornell's response (scratching the medial aspect of the foot beside the extensor tendon of the great toe), and Hirschberg's sign (adduction of the foot on scraping the medial border of the sole).

Looking sideways. *Medical Monitor*, 4 September 1992

Euphuism

Byzantine prose created by doctors striving for literary effect. *See* Decorated Municipal Gothic.

The neurologist with all of his knowledge of minutest anatomy was for years, "like the man who stood on the bridge at midnight", not dreaming the dreams of a Longfellow but soliloquising after the manner of the cynic on the vanity of all earthly things when the voice of the syphilographer first cried out from the darkness "Fear not for I am always with you".

In: Medical pudder. *Res Medica*, Summer 1968

European medicine

1. (Britain) Medicine practised beyond the channel tunnel.

These figures show the incidence is exactly the same in England as it is in Europe.

British anaesthetist addressing European Society of Anaesthesiologists. Brussels, 1993. (He seemed genuinely puzzled when the audience burst into laughter.)

2. (United States) Primitive practices pursued on the other side of the Atlantic.

At a college "mini-course" in Atlanta the chairman, Dr Burton E Bert Sobel, restricted the time allowed to Peter Sleight and hinted that the ISIS data had come from a rather primitive corner of the planet. Peter Sleight responded with the traditional eccentricity expected of an Oxford professor. He appeared at the lectern without his shoes and socks and explained he was a visiting European "barefoot doctor".

Battle of the clotbusters. *BMJ*, 25 May 1991

Evidence based medicine

Perpetuating other people's mistakes instead of your own. *See* Clinical experience.

Expert

Someone who comes from another place and brings **slides**.

Faith

1. What patients expect doctors to have in their treatment.

Over the past month I've been asked did I believe—not had I examined the evidence but did I believe—in copper bracelets for rheumatism, natural childbirth, coronary bypass surgery, and a future for Manchester City. Only the question about Manchester City was acceptable. Football long ago ceased to be a game and became a source of doctrinal dispute, largely because the participants share an unquestioning belief in the power of good and evil. When the lads do well, it is because they believe in themselves. When they do badly, it is the work of the devil. In the words of the liturgy, the score, the referee's decision, or the referee himself was diabolical.

Body and soul. *Guardian*, August 1984

2. A valuable ally in achieving a "cure" and a dangerous enemy in assessing it. *See* Placebo.

Exaggerated claims for the efficacy of a medicament are very seldom the consequence of any intention to deceive; they are usually the outcome of a kindly conspiracy in which everybody has the very best intentions. The patient wants to get well, his physician wants to have made him better, and the pharmaceutical company would like to have put it into the physician's power to have made him so. The controlled clinical trial is an attempt to avoid being taken in by this conspiracy of good will.

P B Medawar.
Advice to a Young Scientist, Harper and Row, 1979

3. A profligate source of self deception.

If there were a verb meaning "to believe mistakenly", it would not have a significant first person, present indicative.

Ludwig Wittgenstein. *Tractatus Logico-Philosophicus*, 1922. Reissued 1949, Routledge and Kegan Paul

Fashion

Powerful influence on medical treatment.

With health, as with clothes, fashion can be set by the famous and the powerful. Define and discuss the influence of Esther Rantzen's pregnancies on attitudes to children and to transplant surgery in Britain of the 1980s. Room there, surely, for a fistful of PhD theses.

The medical condition. *The Listener*, 12 May 1988

In France the ideal bust measurement is 33 inches, in Italy 39. Breasts reduced by surgeons in France would be treasured by Italians. As a result, in Italy, breast augmentation is performed twice as often as breast reduction. In France reduction is almost four times more common than augmentation.

The symptomatology of European chauvinism.
Yorkshire Medicine, Spring 1994

Fashionable doctor

What every private practitioner should strive to become. A doctor to whom the rich and powerful turn instinctively for advice. *See* Harley Street doctor.

> The status is not easily won. You will need to cultivate the interest of gossip columnists—best done by feeding them "off the record" gossip about your patients, sit solemnly through boring luncheons and dinners in the City, and lose no opportunity to hint that yours is an international and aristocratic clientele.
>
> Body and soul. *Guardian*, February 1986

> While you are talking to a patient your secretary enters timidly.
> "Lord Podagra is on the telephone again".
> "Oh, tell him to go to the Devil", and you resume your conversation with a patient who by now is goggling with admiration.
> Some patients might find this method frightening and a more friendly version of the gambit is worth knowing.
> Enter timid (carefully rehearsed) secretary, as before.
> "Excuse me, sir, but his Excellency, the Node of Tawara is on the telephone".
> With a muttered word of excuse you seize your telephone and burst out with: "Hello, Noddy old man. In trouble again? That's too bad".
>
> Richard Asher. Medical salesmanship.
> *Middlesex Hospital Medical Journal*, February 1960

> A fashionable surgeon, like a pelican, can be recognised by the size of his bill.
> J Chalmers da Costa. *The Trials and Triumphs of the Surgeon*, WB Saunders, 1923

Fear

Management technique imported into NHS in the 1990s.

> Recently I sat at dinner between a senior nurse and a senior NHS manager, and much of the talk was of Stalinism in the NHS. These people were convinced that the NHS was becoming an organisation in which people were terrified to speak the truth. This opinion is heard time and time again, and everybody seems convinced that it is becoming worse.
>
> Richard Smith, editor of the BMJ.
> The rise of Stalinism in the NHS. *BMJ*, 17 December 1994

> I am getting a steady flow of correspondence and personal communications from doctors who are scared stiff to be identified. They are unhappy about being instructed to give clinical priority to minor cases over more serious ones to make statistics look good, keep waiting lists down, and give priority to fundholding patients.
>
> Sandy Macara, chairman of BMA Council.
> Quoted in Secrecy in the NHS. *BMJ*, 22 October 1994

> Dr John Spencer, consultant radiologist at Luton and Dunstable Hospital NHS Trust, took early retirement in April 1994 after discovering that the trust's chief executive had tapped his telephone. He signed an agreement not to speak publicly about the circumstance surrounding his retirement.
>
> Naomi Craft.
> Secrecy in the NHS. *BMJ*, 17 December 1994

Feel Good Factor

A sense of blind euphoria induced by large doses of public relations data. Overdosage during the 1980s led to widespread drug resistance and the emergence in the 1990s of a rebound Feel Bad Factor.

Fellowship

Sexist job description still popular in academia. Attracts paradoxical adjectives.

Travelling fellow—One who goes to another place and stays put.
Resident fellow—One appointed to a specific place but who
constantly travels.

Visiting fellow—A travelling fellow who has arrived and does
the work of the resident fellows who are away travelling.

FHSAspeak

A form of **Trustspeak**, which has evolved in new style general
practice.

> Our implicit standards were confounded by retrospective
> analysis resulting in our outcome measures being invalid
> thereby blocking our impetus for change.
>
> *Report on an audit of surgery appointments sent to the*
> *Barnet Medical Audit Advisory Group, 1994*

Gordon Barclay, a GP who became medical advisor to an
FHSA, has compiled a guide to the language he has had to
learn.

Have a meaningful exchange of view	Discuss
Suffer from negative growth	Make a loss
Look at the whole range	Ask someone's advice
No time scale	Never
Flag-up	Tell
Ball park figure	Guess
I will get back to you	Forget it
This needs a fundamental review	No
What are the ramifications?	How much will it cost?
Bring up to speed	Do what I want
They need to understand	Do what I say
Can I clarify what you are saying?	Here are my ideas
I think what you are saying...	Here are my ideas
I think what you are meaning...	Here are my ideas
You are looking at process too soon	You don't agree with me
	Talk through these issues
	Agree with me
Need to get a steer on this	Find people who agree with me
Informal sounding board	I will find people who agree with me.

Monitor Weekly, 29 March and 17 May 1995

Filthy language

Simple Anglo-Saxon words contaminated with an ill understood infection that deters even doctors from using them.

When Eric Partridge wrote *Origins* in 1958 he replaced the central vowels of the two most familiar four letter words with asterisks and wrote: "Outside medical and other learned papers they cannot be printed in full".

Forty years on both those Anglo-Saxon words are often printed in full in the most prestigous of public prints yet medical authors rely on euphemistic verbs of Latin derivation like defecate, micturate, and copulate.
Medical Monitor, 3 April 1996

The stigma of filth is attached to words in an irrational and capricious way. People who shrink from the vulgar will happily use "poppycock" as a form of respectable, gentle swearing. But poppycock derives from the Danish "pappe-kak", which means soft dung. It is said that terse Saxon expressions are no longer used in learned writings because they sound ugly; yet "folk" and "luck", similar in sound to one "obscene" word, are not usually thought to be ugly. It is an emotional revulsion which bans the use of "dirty" words, and this is eventually passed on to the various euphemisms which are used as substitutes.
C Mawdsley. Medical pudder. *Res Medica*, Summer 1968

Dear Sir, You criticise a journalist for using the word c*** on television but, thanks to the euphemistic use of asterisks in your condemnation, we don't know if the word he used was c*** or c***.
Letter to *Independent*, 1988

Flexible

The only adjective ambitious doctors should apply to their beliefs.

Yesterday's dogma is particularly dangerous in medicine. These days to gain acceptance as a progressive obstetrician you need to campaign for more home confinements, to disparage epidural anaesthesia as a grossly overused interference with a natural process, and condemn bottle feeding as a monstrosity almost as grave as infanticide.

Yet just over 20 years ago a progressive obstetrician was expected to abuse reactionaries who criticised plans to have all women delivered in "safer" hospital beds, and had to champion every woman's right to painless childbirth and to free herself from the tyranny of breast feeding.
The flexible dogma game. *An Insider's Guide to the Games Doctors Play*, Gollancz, 1986

Folk remedies

Treatments in which the placebo effect is reinforced by the nostalgia effect, thanks to ingredients that romantics believe were universally available in a bygone rustic age.

For those who find nightmares even more alarming and bizarre than real life, the young tops of the greater periwinkle can be boiled and eaten. When chewed, the leaves also calm nervous disorders and hysteria.
Robin Page. *The Country Way of Cures and Remedies*, Davis-Poynter 1978

No herb ever cures anything, it is only said to cure something. This is always based on the testimony of somebody called Cuthbert who died in 1678. No one ever says what he died of.
Miles Kington. *Nature Made Ridiculously Simple*, 1983. Quoted in *Oxford Dictionary of Humorous Quotations*. 1995

Once upon a time in a touring repertory company, one of the character actors told another that he thought he had piles. Whereupon the second passed on a remedy that had been used in his family for countless generations.

Every morning and every evening, the patient had to make a strong pot of tea, drink three cupfuls, then remove the tea leaves from the pot and pack them tightly in and around his anus.

The actor tried the remedy for five days but his symptoms if anything got worse so he decided to consult a doctor.

An avuncular GP examined him carefully then told him to get dressed. When the patient had resettled himself uneasily in his chair, the doctor spoke: "I have two bits of news. First, I can confirm you have piles. And, second, you are going on a long journey".

Medical Monitor, 21 September 1995

Fountain pen

Despite the advent of computers, remains the Instrument of First Resort in general practice. Largely because those who seek to enrich themselves in the **internal market** have rediscovered high productivity techniques pioneered in the 1950s and '60s by "Wee Willie" McAnny and other Slagthorpe GPs. *See* Scruffie's Triangle.

> Wee Willie's first phase weapon was a large fountain pen with a good reservoir of bright blue Quink and a wide free-flowing nib that allowed it to glide across the surface of certificates and prescriptions like an America's Cup contender on a broad reach.
>
> He knew his patients would feel deprived if they left his premises without a prescription but kept his drug costs well below the average by confining his prescribing to two preparations.
>
> Patients whose symptoms were above their diaphragms got Mist. Tuss. Nig., a black cough mixture whose colour and smell gave it powerful medicinal qualities. Patients with symptoms below the diaphragm got Mist. Mag. Carb Aromat., a white "stomach mixture" whose power lay in its unfailing ability to provoke a satisfactory belch. To maximise throughput, Willie minimised writing time and indicated to the local chemist which preparation should be dispensed by writing just "supra" or "infra" on the prescription.
>
> Looking backwards. *Daily Telegraph*, 26 May 1989

> Today he would top any league table based on cost efficiency, for his methods had the simplicity of genius. They were precisely tailored to the needs of the market and lie waiting to be rediscovered by the next generation of fundholders.
>
> He had, of course, to work hard—he was a martyr to writer's cramp—but he was a kindly man and the punters loved him. Indeed 'twas said around Slagthorpe that all his patients died happy. Young, maybe, but happy.
>
> *Audiomonitor*, January 1997

> An oft-forgotten attribute of clocks is that, if you push the hands forward too far and too fast, you discover you have actually pushed them back.
> Looking backwards. *Daily Telegraph*, 26 May 1989

Function

Any meeting to which a **local medical society** has invited an **expert**.

> My train had arrived one hour late and I was near to running when I burst into the foyer of the small provincial hotel. The receptionist, I remember, sat behind her desk cleaning the dirt from beneath her fingernails with a long plastic knitting needle.
> "Which way to the Balaclava Suite?" I asked.
> "You can't go in there", she said. "There's a function on".
> I heard my voice proclaim a line of stunning pomposity.
> "I am the function".
> A sort of vagrancy. *An Insider's Guide to the Games Doctors Play*, Gollancz, 1986

Functional

Condition often diagnosed in patients referred to hospital for reassurance—of patient or GP or both.

> They receive the fashionable investigations of the day and all too often, in a brief interview, are told that all the results are normal and that there is nothing wrong with them. They are then sent home with a pat on the back, a large bottle of tranquillisers and the symptoms with which they were originally referred. The doctor has never paused to listen to them.
> One feels that often the outcome would be more satisfactory if the doctor and not the patient took the tranquilliser.
> The doctor, the patient, and the tranquilliser. *The Practitioner*, 1964

> Mrs G, a middle class housewife aged thirty eight, managed

to visit her doctor twenty seven times in the course of 10 months. Her three main symptoms were lassitude, a sore throat and a stiff neck. She was referred to a consultant physician, an ear, nose and throat surgeon and an orthopaedic surgeon and was treated for a minor degree of anaemia, chronic pharyngitis and a cervical disc lesion. She had two blood counts, an x ray of her chest and another of her cervical spine. At the end of 10 months she was really no better than she was at the beginning, and her doctor's notes read: "Functional disability. Advised to go on holiday". This advice was no doubt designed primarily for his own relief rather than for that of the patient.

In fact, Mrs G did not go on holiday. She moved house and, because of this, saw another doctor. He looked after her for two years and in that time she visited him only twice. On her first visit his notes read: "Sore throat and stiff neck. Sleeps badly. Before marriage had an illegitimate child. Adopted. Two children of present marriage. Has never told husband. Parents knew. Both dead. They advised against telling husband. Great emotional release in telling story. Treatment nil. Just listened. No advice given". Her second visit was a week later. The doctor's notes read: "Told husband. He knew already. Never felt better in her life".

Ibid

Gait

Funny walks. Much studied by neurologists but sadly neglected by sociologists.

Top end of the social scale, people walk as though they aren't walking anywhere in particular, bottom end of the scale, people walk as though they only had one destination.

Bottom end, people walk as though the movement were being rented rather than owned outright, top end walks are always freehold.

Bottom end walks are really forms of marching, top end people walk as though walking wasn't anything they'd ever had any reason to perfect.

I once saw the late Duke of Marlborough walking up the stairs at Christie's and he did it as though if the legs he was using turned out not to suit him he could get dozens more where they came from.

You can no more disguise your walk than you can your handwriting: I knew a ballet critic who'd once been a policeman, and he always walked up the aisle at Covent Garden as though he were going to take Giselle's name and address.

Robert Robinson. *The Dog Chairman*, Allen Lane, 1982

A family in Grassendale Park made a claim for Disability Living Allowance on behalf of a nine month old baby on the grounds of "inability to walk". Our practice earned £16.40 from the DSS for giving a professional opinion that the child's disability would be likely to improve with the passage of time.

John Winter, Liverpool GP.
Medical Monitor, 17 November 1993

Galileo, Galilei

Dangerous subversive whose record of challenging authority doesn't appeal to many doctors who feel more comfortable with the inductive approach of his contemporary **Francis Bacon**.

Galileo recognised there were usually competing explanations for a phenomenon and tried to devise tests to discriminate between possibilities...

The deductions from a mathematical formula or a hypothesis were subjected to an ordeal; if they failed the test, the experimenter devised fresh experiments in the light of what had already been observed.

This method of discovery depended, as it does today, on an essential element—the creative imagination of the experimenter. It was accepted that the concept of "knowing" has a provisional quality; there is uncertainty about the durability of explanations. And it followed that there must be tentative acceptance of only those theories which have survived rigorous critical tests.

William A Silverman. *Human Experimentation: A Guided Step into the Unknown*, Oxford University Press, 1985

Generalists

Doctors who treat what they assume you have. As opposed to **specialists** who assume you have what they treat. No longer as generalist as they used to be.

> *Sign outside the house of a 19th century English surgeon-apothecary:*
> I Popjay, Surgeon, Apothecary and Midwife, etc.; draws teeth and bleeds on lowest terms. Confectionery, Tobacco, Snuff, Tea, Coffee, Sugar and all sorts of perfumery sold here. N.B. New laid eggs every morning by Mrs Popjay.
> Edward Shorter.
> *Companion Encyclopaedia of the History of Medicine,* In: *Medical Monitor,* 11 June 1997

General public (BMAspeak)

Real people. Not doctors. Also known as "the public at large". *See* Laity.

Geriatric Problem, the

Pejorative phrase used by clinicians and administrators who like to see hospital beds occupied by young people. Better defined as the difficulty old people encounter in getting the care they need.

> Despite a statement by the Royal College of Physicians that the withholding of cardiological investigation and treatment from patients on the grounds of age alone cannot be justified on clinical grounds, a recent survey has shown that a fifth of coronary care units have an upper age limit for admission and two fifths have one for thrombolytic therapy. Discrimination on the grounds that older patients do less well after physiologically challenging interventions is unscientific and inequitable. Age can have no directly causative relationship with outcome. Not every old person shows significant defects and the best approach is to assess each person as an individual.
> J Grimley Evans. *Future trends in medicine,* Royal Society of Medicine, 1993

71

Gideon, doing a

Countering loneliness or depression by reading a familiar text. Named after the Gideon Society that places bibles in hotel rooms.

> A British cardiologist attending a conference in Atlanta flicked idly through the pages of the Gideon Bible in his hotel room and found two 20 dollar bills tucked between the pages. Clipped to them was a note: "If you opened this book because you're discouraged, read the 14th Chapter of John. If you're broke and this would help, take it. If you've had a fight with your wife, buy her a present".
> The message was signed: "A Wayfaring Stranger".
> Beneath it, was a PS. "On second thoughts, maybe you should take it down to the Lotus Room and try their martinis. That's where I got this idea".
> Looking sideways. *Medical Monitor*, 28 August 1992

Gist

What clinical abstracts claim to provide but rarely do. A concept difficult to grasp by medical politicians and the Irish.

> At the annual meeting of the Irish Medical Association, a country GP gave a long, complicated, though highly entertaining, account of some political happening .
> "Excuse me interrupting", said the chairman, "But we're pushed for time. Could you just give us the gist". The speaker looked up angrily. "It's all gist", he said.
> *Monitor Weekly*, 8 June 1994

Glasgow

Enigmatic source of medical wisdom.

> What Glasgow says today the rest of the world tries to understand tomorrow.
> Kenneth Calman. GMC meeting, November 1993

GMC (General Medical Council)

19th Century institution desperately trying to drag itself into the 20th century while there's still time.

GMCspeak

Euphemisms used by the GMC to enable them to discipline doctors without antagonising the trade unionists at the BMA. *See* Performance, Pursuing an improper sexual relationship.

God

Role to which doctors are forever being told they aspire.

> The only doctor I know who really wanted to play God was the physician superintendent of a large asylum in the West Riding of Yorkshire in the 1930s. One day he travelled to Leeds, went to Roundhay Park, rowed himself out to the centre of the lake, and went for a walk on the water.
> When rescued by an off-duty policeman he is alleged to have said: "I fear administration has gone to my head".
> *Medical Monitor*, 15 January 1993

> Clinicians can succumb to flattery from sycophantic patients and begin to wonder whether a divine spark doesn't after all flicker somewhere about their person. But clinical medicine is a great leveller and the evening when you try on the divine robes for size will likely be followed by the morning after when the patient you confidently diagnosed as having acute cholecystitis will produce the mocking rash that heralds shingles.
> One man's burden. *BMJ*, 3 August 1985

> A small boy, treated at Poole General Hospital, is convinced that his tonsils were removed by the Almighty.
> "I was taken into a big room where there were two lady angels and two men angels all dressed in white. One of the men angels looked down my throat and said, 'God, look at this boy's tonsils'.
> And He did".
> *Monitor Weekly*, 23 June 1993

"Whence come disease and healing?" asked the Prophet Moses of God.

"From me", was the reply.

"What purpose then do doctors serve?"

"They earn their living and cultivate hope in the heart of the patient until I either take away his life or give him back his health".

Thus it was written in Nozhat el Majalis.

Alberto Denti di Pirajno. *A Cure for Serpents: An Italian Doctor in North Africa*, Andre Deutsch, 1955

Going for gold

Medical slang for emigrating to the United States.

Americans find it difficult to understand that a doctor should give up medicine to do something else. To them it's like someone handing in the keys to Fort Knox.

World At One. BBC Radio 4, November 1984

An American cardiac surgeon who flew recently from New York to London on Concorde took his seven year old son with him for a treat. As they settled into their seats the boy looked around and asked: "Daddy, what are all these people doing on your plane?"

Anecdotal evidence. *Healthcare Management*, June 1995

The American researcher Allen Roses said that if I re-examined the Statue of Liberty I would see an ancillary inscription: "Send me your trained and underfunded".

Medical Monitor, 22 June 1994

Good old days

An era when doctors knew what was best for their patients.

There is no doubt in my mind that this patient should have termination of pregnancy and sterilisation, not only in her own interests because she is depressed and is unable to cope, but also on eugenic grounds. Continual breeding from such stock is one way of committing racial suicide.

Letter from gynaecologist at Cheltenham General, Eye And Children's Hospital, 1958

(Found in a patient's notes by Dr K R Clarkson.)

In 1945 the *Lancet* feared for the unnatural loss of virginity in British women [using menstrual tampons] so the General Medical Council enforced the printing of the words "unsuitable for unmarried women" on every box.

Caroline White. *BMJ*, 19 January 1991

Dr Chris Scott of Exmouth, searching through a patient's notes, found this letter written by a consultant in 1945.
Poor little Miss L...! I quite agree with you that although she is only 39 she looks much more; but, she looks bereft of all attributes both physical and mental with which a stable person is endowed.

Physically she is underweight, flat bosomed and tight lipped with a large cross on her chest. Mentally, she has always been a weakling ever since she can remember, and has never been quite as strong "in her nerves" as other people.

She represents very typically what is known as a constitutional inferior.

At this age you will be able to do nothing for it whatever, except to give her encouragement and persuasion. I put her on to a simple routine treatment and gave her as much encouragement as possible.

Try, if you can, to keep her off all active treatment, as it is only trying to convert her into something she can never be.

Dr Scott says that 50 years later Poor little Miss L... is "hale and hearty", lives independently at home, and has seen her GP only three times in the past five years.

Medical Monitor, 1 November 1995

Gravitas

Public relations substitute for wisdom. Public demeanour adopted in middle life by doctors with political or academic ambition.

A group of us recently fell to discussing the startling change that occurs in the demeanour of a clever male doctor when the Young Turk transmutes into the Old Fart. Those of you over 40 will recognise the symptoms. Men who once were lively, witty and intelligent companions suddenly assume a public persona quite at odds with the character that previously served them well.

Where once they would have enlivened conversation,

they make observations of paralysing ordinariness. And, on the slightest of excuses, they will rise to their feet to make pompous speeches. Drawn into public discussion, they rasp on earnestly and nod wisely as if naught but weighty thoughts were granted admission to their minds. Most grievously of all, they refrain from using their private wit in public places for fear that amusing or penetrating remarks might prove "politically inept".

Anecdotal evidence. *Medical Interface*, December 1995

Develops inevitably into **pomposity**, the unavoidable fate of those who believe that in order to be seen to be serious, they need to be seen to be solemn.

You must not think me necessarily foolish because I am facetious...nor will I comprehend you necessarily wise because you are grave.

Sidney Smith. In: One man's burden.
BMJ, 21 October 1983

Make him laugh and he will think you a trivial fellow, but bore him in the right way and your reputation is assured.

W Somerset Maugham.
Gentleman in the Parlour, Heinemann, 1930

Gravitas, the heavy tread of moral earnestness, becomes a bore if it is not accompanied by the light step of intelligence.

The Listener, 20 March 1969

Grey Suits

People whose clothing reflects their state of mind. Ill assorted collection of company directors, accountants, management consultants, and other commissioned officers in the "market forces" who have taken positions of power in the NHS.

A civilised society is one in which businessmen, like soldiers, are on tap, not on top. The idea that the finance director of a ball-bearing firm should be in a position to determine the surgical priorities of a hospital, the programme of a theatre or the curriculum of a university is, a priori, absurd. Yet such absurdities routinely occur in contemporary Britain as public bodies continue to be packed with government nominees drawn from the business sector.

[One] reason why businessmen should not be allowed to dominate public bodies is...that most businessmen are ignorant. If you think that this admirably qualifies them to represent the general public, pause for a moment. While you or I might feel humbled by our ignorance, the businessman feels no such diffidence, for he does know about the only thing which apparently matters, namely the "bottom line".

John Naughton. Crawling along the bottom line.

Observer, 7 January 1996

Health Minister Gerry Malone has issued a press statement welcoming the new chairman of the Guy's and St Thomas' NHS Trust, Sir Kenneth Eaton.

Having listed the areas in which the trust is regarded as a centre of excellence—they include cardiology, dermatology, foetal medicine, and neurology—Mr Malone describes the new chairman's unique qualification for the job. "His last five years were spent in charge of the Trident submarine programme".

Monitor Weekly, 21 June 1995

Group therapy

Psychiatry's contribution to increased productivity. One psychiatrist assembles a bunch of patients and sits and listens while they treat one another.

In more progressive trusts the psychiatrist only pretends to listen while making notes about more urgent matters like shortfall control, clinical throughput, and the department's business plan.

Grundyism

A depressing eagerness, on the part of doctors, to issue warnings about activities they see other people enjoying. *See* Masturbation.

Hazards published in learned journals include: jogger's nipple, break-dancer's neck, crab-eater's lung, swim-goggle headache, amusement slide anaphylaxis, cyclist's pudendum, dog walker's elbow, space invaders' wrist, unicyclist's sciatica, jeans folliculitis, jogger's kidney, flautist's neuropathy, and urban cowboy's rhabdomyolosis—a painful nastiness in the muscles caused by riding mechanical bucking broncos in amusement arcades.

Three punctilious Swiss, Drs Itin, Heanel, and Stalder, from Kantonsspital Liestal, reported yet another jogging hazard: bird attacks by the European buzzard (*Buteo buteo*). The attacks occur during the buzzard breeding season and "the birds attacked by diving from behind and continuing to dive as long as the joggers were in motion". Sadly the good doctors didn't speculate on what was passing through the buzzards' minds at the time.

There's a doctor close behind you. *An Insider's Guide to the Games Doctors Play*, Gollancz, 1986

Old men give young men good advice, no longer being able to give them bad example.

C E M Joad.
Trasymachus, or the future of morals, Kegan Paul 1925

Cycling

If the pedals are too far from the seat, the rider cannot make her feet follow the pedals without inclining the pelvis. Such side to side movement of the pelvis produces unnecessary strain on the muscles of the back and loins, and also friction against the sensitive external genitals. If the saddle is badly shaped, the friction thus produced may lead to bruising, even to excoriations, and short of this, in women of certain temperament, to other effects on the sexual system, which we need not particularise.

Dr Herman. *BMJ*, 1895

There must be few of us who have not seen the ill effects of over-exertion on a bicycle. The commonest is palpitation and temporary dilatation but even this is sometimes very difficult to cure...that temporary dilatation occurs is enough to show the great strain put upon the heart, and it is an added danger that the sense of fatigue in the limbs is so slight. The rider is thus robbed of the warning to which he is accustomed to attend, and repeats or continues the strain upon the heart. As in other similar cases, the effect is to render that dilatation permanent which was at first but temporary, and to cause an increase in the muscle of the heart by repeated exertion. The heart produced is of large dimensions and of thick walls—a condition which may, perhaps, give little uneasiness to its owner, but which a medical man will view with considerable distrust and apprehension.

Leading article. *BMJ*, 1898

Eighteen years ago, when 35 years of age, the writer was among the first to adopt the bicycle as a means of recreation. For some six years I rode the high wheel, usually devoting the month of August to a tour of several hundred miles. The saddles at that time, and for years afterward, were unsanitary and injurious in their effects because of the pressure against the perineum, and the consequent irritation of the prostate gland. As the riding was at that time largely confined to young men, the results of the unsanitary saddles, rigid frames and excessive vibration were scarcely realised even by the medical profession. What these consequences have been to many men, it required the later years to disclose.

Sylvanus Stall. *What a Man of Forty-five Ought to Know*, VIR Publishing, 1901

Kissing

The dangers of kissing include the transmission of scurvy, diphtheria, herpes, parasitic diseases, ringworm, and ulcerative stomatitis....One person kissed on the ear suffered a rupture of the eardrum undoubtedly due to suction...frequent kissing of children can induce precocious puberty, undue excitement of sexual organs, and irregular menstruation.

Samuel Adams.
Journal of the American Medical Association, 1886

In 1993, five Finnish doctors, writing in the *Lancet*, warned against kissing Russian girls, as one tourist (among some 400 000 Finns who visit Russia every year) returned from St Petersburg with diphtheria. Though he admitted that he had kissed a girl, he had also drunk from unwashed glasses at a birthday party. The local girl remained healthy, but the doctors believed that "contact with a local inhabitant" was of public health importance.

Petr Skrabanek. *The Death of Humane Medicine and the Rise of Coercive Healthism*, The Social Affairs Unit, 1994

Guarded

Pathologically uncommitted.

> Dr C N Faulkes of Letchworth found this note from Social
> Services in the folder of a 88 year old patient: "His form of
> leukaemia is, as I say, chronic, and he has had it now for
> over eight years. His ultimate prognosis must be guarded in
> view of his age".
>
> *Monitor Weekly*, 12 April 1995

Harley Street doctor

Postgraduate qualification that demands no attributes or skills
other than renting a room in right location. Since 1920s has been
useful qualification for doctors who specialise in diseases of the
rich. *See* Legacy doctors.

> Most of these patients were women, many of them rich,
> idle, spoiled, and neurotic. I was firm, I was stern, I bullied
> and commanded, I even invented a new disease for them—
> asthenia. This word became a sort of talisman, which
> procured my entry to more important portals. At afternoon
> tea in Cadogan Place, or Belgrave Square, Lady Blank
> would announce to the Honourable Miss Dash—eldest
> daughter of the Earl of Dot:
> "Do you know, my dear, this young Scottish doctor—
> rather uncivilised, but amazingly clever—has discovered
> that I'm suffering from asthenia. Yes, asthenia. And for
> months old Dr Brown Blodgett kept telling me it was
> nothing but nerves".
>
> A J Cronin. *Adventures in Two Worlds*, Gollancz, 1952
>
> Having created a disease, it was essential to produce the
> remedy. Again and yet again my sharp and shining needle
> sank into fashionable buttocks, bared upon the finest linen
> sheets. I became expert, indeed, superlative, in the art of
> penetrating the worst end of the best society with a dexterity
> which rendered the operation almost painless.
> Strange though it may seem, the results of this complex

process of hocus-pocus—and I was, I assure you, a great rogue at this period, though perhaps not more so than many of my colleagues—were surprisingly, often amazingly, successful. Asthenia gave these bored and idle women an interest in life. My tonics braced their languid nerves. I dieted them, insisted on a regime of moderate exercise and early hours. I even persuaded two errant wives to return to their long-suffering husbands and, within nine months, they had matters other than asthenia to occupy them.

Ibid

Health

1. Ill defined entity on sale in urban High Streets where health food shops, sports couturiers, and "work out" parlours proliferate with an exuberance that indicates real money is changing hands.

> It's not surprising people grow confused and start to think that to be healthy you've got to suffer, give up things you enjoy, become a food faddist or, even worse, the sort of exercise freak who equates health with physical fitness and ends up Mens Insana in Corporate Sauna.
> Health, wealth, and happiness.
> *The Listener*, 30 October 1989

> Irma Kurtz recognised the self centred character of the new health religion. Writing in the *Journal of Medical Ethics* she described it as a paltry faith which has nothing to do with improving the lot of one's fellow men, but which worships only Self.
> Petr Skrabanek. *The Death of Humane Medicine and the Rise of Coercive Healthism*, The Social Affairs Unit, 1994

2. Vital personal attribute under constant threat from hazards eagerly reported by the media.

> So many things in this world can damage our health, it's a wonder that any of us get out of it alive.
> Sir Richard Doll. *Can you avoid cancer?* BBC TV, 1984

> Woman overheard on American radio: "I read this article. It said the typical symptoms of stress are eating too much, smoking too much, impulse buying, and driving too fast.

Are they kidding? This is my idea of a great day".
                                                    Anecdotal evidence.
                                    Healthcare Management, August 1994

Card handed to all visitors arriving in Taiwan:
"Welcome! We hope your visit will be a pleasant one.
Should you become ill during your stay in Taiwan within six
weeks (symptoms of vomiting, diarrhea, chill and fever,
headache, general muscles soreness, arthralgia, skin rash,
cough, night sweating, dramatic decrease of body weight or
enlargement of lymph node, etc,) you may have infected
with communicable diseases.

In order to prevent yourself and your neighbourhood who
might be infected from you by secondary transmission,
please carry this card and contact the nearest health
station".
Someone should have added: "Have a nice day".
                                    Monitor Weekly, 22 March 1995

3. A fantasy defined by the World Health Organization: "A state
of complete physical, mental, and social wellbeing".

I reckon we're lucky we achieve that state at occasional
moments in our lifetimes. Most of us for most of the time
have some niggle or ache, some twinge of anxiety or
depression, which we accept as part of the business of being
alive.
                                    Body and soul. *Guardian*, June 1984

4. A subject on which **educationalists** like to exercise their
vocabulary.

Health and "disease" are normative concepts. That is to say,
they are polar terms in a continuum between optimum
functioning and malfunctioning of an organism. When we
consider the World Health Organization definition of health,
"complete physical, mental, and social wellbeing...and not
just the absence of disease", we are clearly dealing with
health as a value concept.
                                                    Ian Thompson.
                        Focus on health, Lothian Health Board, May 1985

5. Displacement activity for obsessionals.

An "intelligent toilet" is being developed in Japan. It
automatically measures indices of health and disease in the

stool and urine, and if the user inserts a finger into a device built into one side of the toilet, it gives an instant record of pulse rate and blood pressure. The spokesman for the research team said: "It is our dream that some day people's homes will be linked via communications lines to a health centre which could monitor the changes in vital signs read by the toilet".

Guardian, 20 October 1989

6. Elusive entity akin to happiness.

As a GP, I saw many of my patients with chronic disabling diseases lead more rewarding—in my book "healthier"—lives than others who knew they were healthy because they'd had the "check-ups" to prove it yet lived in uneasy conflict with the world around them.

Looking sideways. *Medical Monitor*, 25 May 1992

Health is that choice seasoning which gives relish to all our enjoyments.

John Morgan, 1765

Health gains

Nonsensical data that allow **accountants** to believe they know what's going on in general practice.

Letter to local GPs from Mr A G Sensicle, Director of Finance of Clwyd FHSA:
Clwyd local health strategies—GP workload analysis
I am seeking to assess each GP's time attributable to the various local health strategy areas.

Where practitioners receive income in respect of areas directly attributable to specific aspects of the contract then this is relatively easily available centrally. Similarly, I can assess prescribing to Health Gain areas via a mapping exercise between PACT chapters and health gain areas. What I do not know is how general medical duties are perceived to be attributable across health gain areas (based on the time content of patient contacts).

Your assistance is requested in relation to: (a) % of your time spent and (b) % of prescriptions issued, for each health gain area.

[Mr Sensicle, you will notice, shows no interest in the %

of your time you'll spend trying to translate his prose.]
You may be able to provide this information in one of the
following ways:
1. Estimate percentages based on personal experience
2. Obtain percentages from computerised or manual
records
3. Record actual information over a two/three week
period.

*The form Mr S provides does not require GPs to indicate
whether the data they supply is estimated or measured so we
can all guess how accurate it will be.*
Medical Monitor, 10 November 1993

Health lobby

Pejorative term used by makers of lethal or dangerous products to
describe busybodies who try to tell consumers about the
dangers.

Health promotion

Good idea given bad name by enthusiasts. Much activity
conducted in its name is based on wishful thinking because
individuals have only a tiny degree of control over their own
health compared with the influence of heredity, culture, environment, and chance.

> The aim of medicine is surely not to make men virtuous; it
> is to safeguard and rescue them from the consequences of
> their vices.
> H L Mencken.
> Quoted in *Healthcare Management*, January 1995

Healthy exercise

Any exercise you enjoy taking.

> Whatever you do, don't force yourself into exercise you
> don't enjoy because you think it is making you healthy.

Health, I'm sure, has more to do with happiness than with unenjoyable activities alleged to produce a mythical "fitness". The myth is summed up in the tale of the "health enthusiast" who, when his friend dropped dead while jogging alongside him, gazed down and said rather proudly: "What a way to go, in the peak of condition".

Executive health, *International Management*, June 1983

Heroic treatment

Phrase much favoured by surgeons. Intended to imply glorious conduct on the part of the surgeon though the heroism is, of course, demanded of the patient.

Heroine addiction

Odd condition induced by tired proof reading.

New aspects of heroine addiction.
AMA Journal, November 1982

I did Joan of Arc in A-level history and it didn't touch me. But when I left school I started to experiment with soft stuff. Angela Rippon's biography, that class of thing. Then one evening I went to *Traviata* and, by the end of act two, I was into the hard stuff.

Within a month I was travelling the country for a fix. *La Boheme* in Glasgow, *Tosca* in Cardiff, then back to the Garden for *Isolde* or *Butterfly*. And all the while I was feeding my daily habit with Catherine Cooksons.

I started trading, knocking off romantic novels and peddling them to raise cash for the hard stuff. One week I unloaded a dozen Claire Rayners and blew my mind on uncut *Brunnhilde* at the Garden: *Walkure*, *Siegfried*, and *Gotterdammerung* one after the other. Man, that was flying.

But once you're into a full Ring cycle, there's no turning back and I woke up in a treatment centre. Replacement therapy. Joyce Grenfell records. Selected tales from *Listen with Mother*. Moments with Ella Wheeler Wilcox.

And now I'm out I want to know, straight up doc, is there any cure?

Not exactly a cure, said the GP handing over a pile of Barbara Cartlands. But take one of these every day till you finish the course. It's what we doctors call aversion therapy.

Looking sideways. *Medical Monitor*, 11 January 1991

High falution

Pseudoprofundity. One way to rise quickly in the medical profession.

Remember that the harder anything is to understand, the more readily will committees allocate money to it. Much sensible medicine is obvious, but the obvious does not impress. If only you will trouble to learn the art of putting obvious or trite things in a quasi-profound way then the world will be at your feet. There is a more or less standard technique for turning the obvious into the profound. It depends largely on using certain key words and expressions as often as you can. Here are the most important ones:

broadly based, dynamic, integrated in perspective, stressor influences, unit, social economic and environmental condition, psycho-social, psycho-biological, psychodynamic (psycho-any thing will do, except psychosomatic which is just a little overdone).

Do not study diseases, but "observe the natural history of the disease". Do not study patients, but "study the whole man" or, better still, "view the individual in perspective against his economic and psycho-social background", or "consider his dynamic status within the group".

Richard Asher. Medical salesmanship.
Middlesex Hospital Medical Journal, February 1960

Hippocrates

Greek physician venerated by those who believe he invested their profession with a religious mystique that it still retains. *See* Aaronical.

Thought to have lived in 5th century BC, though no one is sure of his dates to within 20 or 30 years. Alleged author of **Hippocratic Oath**. (Some scholars claim that none of the texts of the Hippocratic corpus, many of which are contradictory, were written by the man after whom they are named.)

> One day in the mid-fifties there was one of those ceremonies the BMA is rather keen on. In the presence of the Greek Ambassador and any number of BMA notables, a distinguished representative of the Greek medical profession planted in Garden Court a small sprig said to have been taken from the very plane tree under which Hippocrates used to sit uttering aphorisms in Cos. Polite applause pattered about the court and garden as the ceremonial sod was lifted and the frail specimen gently placed in the alien soil, symbolising the handing on of a centuries-old tradition, a noble ideal for the BMA to guard. The cutting died within a few weeks.
>
> Mr Hyde. *World Medicine*, 11 July 1973

Hippocratic Oath

Catalogue of restrictive practices dressed up as a solemn promise to Apollo. An oath invoked more often than it is sworn.

> It takes little consideration of the Hippocratic Oath to conclude that it is a bigoted and dangerous document. It embraces hard-line early trade union practices, including the closed family shop, intended to establish a mystery about the men who practised the art which would separate them from other beings. As well as encouraging nepotistic incompetent hierarchies, it hands out totally ambiguous ethical advice.
>
> Robert Reid. *World Medicine*, 11 July 1973

> Contrary to popular belief, the Hippocratic Oath is no fixed and unalterable document of medical ethics, but has been constantly modified over the centuries. Nor was it ever widely sworn or imposed as a condition for obtaining a degree or entering practice. The earliest certain evidence for the Oath taken in a university comes from 1558, and not until 1804 is there evidence for it being sworn by graduands or students. The demand for medical oaths and declarations is largely a feature of the second half of the twentieth century, favoured by physicians but often viewed with suspicion by patients.
>
> Vivian Nutton. *What's in an oath?*
> Lecture at Royal College of Physicians, 25 July 1995

Hip replacement

New NHS unit of currency. Health Ministers justifying increased prescription charges now say, "This will allow us to do x thousand more hip replacements" when once they would have said "This will allow us to build x new hospitals".

The new currency unit has a lot going for it. To the non-participant it is an easily definable operation that allows elderly cripples to walk again and avoids the complex mess you get into when you try to define, say, cancer treatment.

Its only snag is that it doesn't convey the reality of the world of market forces. It would be truer to say: "This will allow us to provide x more cars for Trust executives ... employ x more public relations consultants for Trust chairmen...be ripped off by x more computer companies...".

Monitor Weekly, 13 April, 1994.

Holistic

Oddly spelt word that appears a lot in the *Guardian*. Coined in the 1920s, to express the notion, long a part of medicine, that doctors should treat each patient as a "whole" person and not as a collection of symptoms.

Sometimes used to defend treatments that can adduce little scientific evidence to support their claims of success but can claim to use a "whole person" approach. Hence:

More holistic than thou
Attitude adopted by purveyors—and consumers—of treatment that can muster little scientific backing and thus appeals to radical instincts. Mutual enthusiasm of purveyors and consumers transmutes the treatment into "a cause", an article of faith to be promulgated with religious fervour and defended vigorously against all criticism regardless of its merit.

Home ground

Uncomfortable place to practice.

John Oldroyd chose to work in the West Riding town in

which he'd grown up. One day at the local hospital he was giving an anaesthetic to a woman and, as he prepared to inject the pentothal, she asked: "Did I hear the nurse call you Dr Oldroyd?"

"Yes", said John.

"So is Mr Oldroyd at the Mill your father?"

"Yes".

The woman smiled wistfully, and before slipping into oblivion, muttered: "You know, if I'd played my cards right I could have been your mother".

Medicine has the last laugh.
BMA News Review, December 1991

Hospice

Archaic institution wholly out of place in market led service. Wastes valuable skills and resources when the only outcome is known to be death.

> If I were asked to name people who in our time have proved worthy successors to William Marsden I would nominate the Sisters of Charity, who founded the first modern hospice for the dying—St Joseph's Hospice in London—and whose ideas were energetically espoused by Dame Cicely Saunders.
>
> When those nuns and Dame Cicely saw there was a group of patients who didn't have the right credentials for our modern metropolitan hospitals, they created hospitals of their own. And, in doing so, started an international movement which has helped remind Western countries that we still need hospitals dedicated simply to caring for people, sustaining their spirit, and relieving their pain. One of the glories of the hospice movement is that the care it offers is founded not just on kindness and good intentions but on scientific knowledge and skill.
>
> Marsden lecture, Royal Free Hospital, 1984

Hospital premises

Photo opportunity sites for politicians.

> Readers of your Godalming editions saw Mrs Bottomley

pictured with my father pulling a Christmas cracker when he was a patient at Milford hospital.

Although described as one of her constituents, he is not her greatest fan (who is?) but nevertheless went along with the photograph. What wasn't told was that it was Mrs Bottomley who insisted on having a "prop".

Nursing staff spent more than 20 minutes touring the hospital to locate a cracker.

Reader's letter. *Surrey Advertiser*, February 4 1995

House names

Cabalistic phrases carved on pieces of wood that the English middle class place in obscure corners of their property to ward off GPs seeking them by torch light on rainy nights.

The specimen names the shop had chosen to exemplify the different styles of carving gave a clue to the sort of customers it dealt with: The Maltings, The Cedars, The Old Rectory. They were all painfully familiar. In my time in general practice, the easiest night calls—in terms of actually finding the patient—were to working class terraced houses that abutted the pavement and had numbers prominently displayed above the door knocker.

The most elusive patients were those who considered it a social necessity to drop the numbers from their homes and give them names.

Monitor Weekly, 14 September 1994

I often got a hint of the sort of people I was going to meet by the degree of pretension in the naming of their homes. One family, for instance, called their house Halton Hall, which, no doubt looked more impressive on their notepaper than on their pebble-dashed semi-detached bungalow.

The only place where people used imagination was the local caravan site. The Macbeths called their caravan Cawdor, the Salt family called theirs The Cruet, and quiet little Mr Twigg, who lived on his own, called his Strangeways Jail. When I asked him why, he said it provoked interesting conversation whenever he had to give his address.

Ibid

Human experimentation

The well intentioned guesswork of everyday practice. Phrase more often used to criticise controlled trials.

Ethical arguments raised when patients are to be allocated to compared treatments take one of two mutually contradictory forms. The first contends that the group receiving standard treatment is sacrificed because they are denied the benefit of a favourable new therapy. The second expresses concern that patients allotted to an untested innovation are exposed to an unwarranted risk.

William A Silverman. *Human Experimentation: A Guided Step into the Unknown*, Oxford University Press, 1985

There is a more urgent need to protect patients from the uncontrolled experimentation which characterises much "accepted medical practice" by altruistic, but scientifically uncritical, clinicians.

Iain Chalmers. *World Medicine*, April 1978

Richard Smithells, Professor of Paediatrics at the University of Leeds, has written: "I need permission to give a drug to half my patients but not to give it to them all".

Executive health. *International Management*, April 1983

Human resources

Trustspeak for "people". The distancing phrase allows managers to regard human beings not as quirky individuals but as commodities or computable items.

When a Birmingham GP, Tony Ball wrote to his local FHSA asking for a definition of "human resource manager" he received this "clarification":

"Human resource management is directed mainly at management needs or human resources (not necessarily employees) to be provided and deployed. There is greater emphasis on planning, monitoring and control, rather than on problem-solving and mediation. It is totally identified with management interests, being a general management activity and is relatively distant from the workforce as a whole".

> Just what we need in medicine. And the more distant the
> better.
>> *Monitor Weekly*, 18 January 1995

Hyperactivity

Antisocial behaviour in one's own children. As opposed to
parental control, lack of: antisocial behaviour in other people's
children.

Hyperexegesis

Syntactical hypertrophy induced by an overeagerness to explain.
See Pedagoguery.

> It sounds as though he has an acute protruding disc and
> perhaps an extruded disc now that the traction seems to have
> aggravated it. This is usually used to distinguish between a
> protruding disc which will not disappear and an extruded
> disc which both would seem to get worse under traction and
> compare that with the usual degenerated bulging disc which
> usually disappears on traction. If this is true, the patient
> should be subjected to myelography and probably the disc
> should be taken out.
>> Neurosurgeon's report quoted by Edmund J Simpson. Verba
>> sesquipedalia. *Journal of the American Medical
>> Association*, 20 January 1969

Iatrogen

The international unit of humility.

Ignorance, feigned

Traditional technique used by medical teachers to maintain
intellectual authority over students and juniors.

The technique of pseudo-ignorance is suitable for elderly men and starts with asking numerous artless questions, rather like certain judges do. "What is this free hydrochloric acid they mention in the report?" or "Let me see now. What are these new fangled anticoagulants everyone is talking about?" and so on.

Then, after carefully building up an impression of helpless senility, you suddenly produce a sparkling, up to date dissertation on the tanned red cell agglutination test for autoimmune thyroid antibodies, revealing a knowledge of the very latest published and even unpublished work. The manoeuvre involves very little strain. You need study only one contemporary discovery fairly thoroughly to make it shine wonderfully against the carefully constructed background of senility.

Richard Asher. Medical salesmanship.
Middlesex Hospital Medical Journal, February 1960

Illness

1. A chunk of someone's life. Sometimes used by people who should know better as a synonym for disease.

Every illness is unique, its nature determined not just by an assault by disease or physical insult but by the mental and physical state of the individual assaulted. The same disease can run such different courses in different people that it sometimes needs different treatment. And a patient's resolution and determination can sometimes have more influence on the course of a illness than high-powered medical technology.

How to Succeed in Business
Without Sacrificing your Health, Gollancz, 1988

2. Sometimes less an evil than an opportunity.

My own experience of the usefulness of illness goes back to childhood. Illness to me brought a comfortable bed, a glowing, flickering fire, and seclusion. I can still recall the impression made on me by the books I read at the time. School reinforced this. Hugh Walpole's Mr Perrin and Mr Trail, read in the sickbay, has since been one of my most vivid memories. So is my stay of three weeks with chickenpox in the sanatorium where my incarceration led me to the first original scientific concept that I formed.

George Pickering.
Creative Malady, George Allen and Unwin, 1974

Image

Most significant characteristic of individuals or institutions in an age more concerned with shadow than with substance.

High on my list of improbable people comes a surgeon worried about his image. Most surgeons with whom I have brushed shoulders have had an enviable air of reliability, self confidence, and *sang froid*— a quality that sounds more flattering in French than in translation.

I suspect that a "good public image" is akin to other abstractions like dignity, a sense of humour, or sex appeal. If you find yourself worrying over whether you've got it, you've probably got something to worry about. These are accolades that other people award you if you are lucky. To try to award them to yourself is to court disaster.

The public image of surgery. Lecture at Royal College of Surgeons in Ireland, February 1984

A group of fund holding GPs in the North East is handing out questionnaires in the hope of discovering how they are "perceived" by their patients. I wonder will the answers be as truthful as that once offered to a Worcester GP.

Visiting a patient at home, he had to pass a deaf old lady sitting in a chair. As he went by, she stared at him with a puzzled frown. "Who's this?" she asked.

"It's the doctor", said her daughter.

"Who?"

"The doctor, mother".

"Who?"

"The doctor", said the daughter, now shouting.

"The what?"

"You know, mother. The man who killed father".

Anecdotal evidence. *Healthcare Management*, May 1993

Someone labelled "a psychologist" appeared on my television screen to explain what he called the decline in medicine's "professional image". Our problem it seems is that we no longer "radiate success".

For a moment I hoped—though in vain—he would

suggest that we follow the advice of Dr Samuel Johnson: "A successful doctor needs three things. A top hat to give him authority; a paunch to give him dignity, and piles to give him an anxious expression".

Anecdotal evidence. *Medical Interface*, January 1997

Impression, making a good

Odd yet lingering tradition of patients putting on "good", sometimes even "best", clothes for a visit to the doctor as if going to church or visiting royalty.

A Glasgow GP, Dr P S Wiggins, spoke of a friend who recently attended her GP for a cervical smear. During the procedure the doctor (male) mentioned, in a kindly way, that she had obviously gone to some trouble to prepare herself. It seemed an unusual comment and, on her way home, she wondered what he meant.

She later mentioned the remark to her daughter explaining that all she'd done before going to the surgery was to have a wash and use her daughter's Fem Fresh spray. Only then did she discover that, by mistake, she had used her daughter's disco glitter.

Monitor Weekly, 13 July 1994

Inconsequentiality

Most attractive feature of general practice.

A book review in the July issue of the *British Journal of General Practice* begins: "One of the greatest frustrations of general practice is its lack of absolutes and certainties".

Funny. I've always thought that was one of its great attractions.

Medical Monitor, 23 August 1995

Despite developments in primary care over the past 40 years an enduring core of general practice remains unchanged. Here are some of the questions patients asked, and comments they made, in a South London surgery in the 1950s and '60s.

I'm glad I've got somebody to console my troubles to.

When you're young they say it's growing pains. What is it when you're old? Shortening pains?

My husband wears a protective but sometimes he forgets himself.

Retirement—They've given me a nice clock to see my time pass away.

Presbyopia—When I thread a needle, I have to look outside of my eye.

Losing weight—We've found a new one, doc. Sex is 200 calories so we're having it eight times a day.

GP to woman in retirement home—Why don't you sit outside in the sunshine on one of the benches?

Woman—Oh, I wouldn't risk it. I don't want to be a poppy show. There's only one from here who does. They call her the News of the World.

Tom Madden. Entries from his notebook quoted in *Medical Monitor*, 22 January and 5 February 1997

Innocence of childhood

Myth fostered by adults who've forgotten how often, and how easily, they manipulated "grown ups" when they themselves were children.

I suppose he was aged about 11 at the time and I was worried that he might have acute appendicitis. True his mother had told me that, despite her warning, he had eaten a bagful of green apples but you all know how dangerous a "green apple" diagnosis can be at that age. As I dithered at the bedside, trying to make a decision, I filled in time by asking him what was so great about green apples.

"I didn't eat them because I liked them", he said haughtily. "I ate them to find out why my mother didn't want me to".

Monitor Weekly, 29 June 1994

Insight

Occasional glimpse that life affords us of not just who but what we are.

Some 30 years ago, as a newly hatched medical journalist,

I made a brief appearance on the BBC's early evening news. The sewer workers were on strike and I was there to reassure the punters that when the sewage seeped up into the streets the main threat would be not to their health but to their aesthetic sensitivity.

As I left Television Centre, an actor friend, then starring in a weekly series, offered me a lift home. And, as we passed through the main gates on our way to the car park, two small boys approached and asked for our autographs. Impressed by the transient fame bestowed by a few authoritative words on sewage, I proudly signed my name. As we walked away, I heard one boy say to his chum: "I got (he mentioned my friend's name). Who did you get?"

The boy whose book I'd signed replied: "A load of old rubbish".

Medical Monitor, 5 February 1997

Internal market

An artificial market created to subject artistic or altruistic endeavours to the discipline of "market forces" otherwise known as unrestrained greed.

> The [old] system worked reasonably well. It was relatively cheap, efficient and helped to make the population healthy. But this was not enough for the idealists of the class of '79. The NHS did not conform to market principles; it was the seat of egalitarian collectivism and as a monopoly it necessarily had to be inefficient. The NHS did not have to compete to provide treatment, it was said; there was no overt pressure in the system to produce at lower cost nor any means by which efficient "producers" could get more business or expand. So the NHS was reinvented as a market, with thinking influenced by failed US theorists who were confronting a genuine crisis in health care costs, as the British were not.
>
> Will Hutton. *The State We're In*, Vintage, 1995

> Far from bringing efficiency, the internal market brought confusion to hospitals already trying to cope with chaos. The medical reaction was summed up in a jaunty graffito I found in a London teaching hospital. At eye level above a urinal in the gents used by doctors I read: *At this moment you're the only man in this hospital who*

97

> *knows what he's doing.*
>
> *Plymouth Medical Society Bicentenary Meeting,*
> April 1994

International medicine

A myth.

> It isn't how sick you are but where you are when you get
> sick that determines how you're treated by a doctor.
>
> *Newsweek*, 26 September 1988

> The overall incidence of heart disease in Germany is the
> same as in Britain yet Germans consume six times more
> heart drugs than Britons and their doctors diagnose
> *Herzinsuffizienz* on grounds that would not lead to a
> diagnosis of heart disease in other European countries....A
> German can enjoy bad health because the acceptable
> national mood is pessimism. A senior businessman will take
> his "heart medicine" publicly and with pride because it
> enhances his status. Britons tend to swallow their tablets in
> secret because the knowledge that they were "flawed" might
> inhibit their advancement.
>
> The French, as every Briton knows, are obsessed with
> their livers. An ingenuous American researcher comparing
> survival rates in intensive care units was alarmed by the
> high death rate attributed to liver disease in France. What he
> was measuring, of course, was the incidence not of the
> disease but of the attribution.
>
> What nationality is your ulcer?
> *Sunday Times Magazine*, August 1989

> You will find that on one side of a frontier cellulitis means
> muscular rheumatism, and on the other it involves purulent
> inflammation of the subcutaneous tissue; a hundred kilo-
> metres further on it is a euphemism for obesity in puffy
> young women.
>
> Dr M N G Dukes. *BMJ*, 1973

> Medical information still has problems crossing national
> boundaries. At a recent meeting of some 300 GPs I asked if
> anyone could give me the name of just one French journal.
> No one could.
>
> The symptomatology of European chauvinism.
> *Rocket*, Spring 1994

Interventionist

Pejorative term used by food manufacturers to describe any member of the **health lobby** who advises people to modify their **traditional British diet.** Doctors who report risks linked to diet are dangerous interventionists; advertising food products with aggressive enthusiasm is not interventionist.

Irritable vowel syndrome

Phonetic uncertainty that afflicts people who migrate to London from the north. Journalist Jill Tweedie confessed that when she came south and was faced with phrases like "dance band" or "Stafford Castle", she could never remember in which word to posh up the vowel sound.

Similar dilemma now faces Trustafarians and other rich young things who seek street credibility by poshing down their vowels.

> An infallible way of diagnosing a Northcountryman who has developed a southern accent is to give him two pints of beer and ask him to say "jam puff".
> Dr M J Streule, Buckinghamshire GP.
> *Personal communication*

Jabberwock Syndrome

Interpretative disorder induced by cutbacks in hospital secretarial services.

> The slithy toves of Gwynedd
> Paul Nickson who practises in Bethesda received this from a local ophthalmology department. "The intraocular pressures were at the top of the normal range and the gonioscopy revealed slightly anemones strange angles with an anterior iris incision, however this unmoral does occur

guise commonly in individuals with out glaucoma".

Medical Monitor, 7 February 1995

From a letter to John Anderson of Sidmouth from an orthopaedic surgeon: "She has some features of Parkinson's disease, namely a bit of trunkle, ataxia, some Cogwell rigidity, and also some rather typical faeces".

Medical Monitor, 15 May 1996

From a letter to Dr Mike Cohen of Aylesbury from Stoke Mandeville Hospital NHS Trust: "I saw X in my clinic. He has a right thumb deviated slightly grip. His urethral opening is terminal".

Well it would be, wouldn't it?

Medical Monitor, 21 September 1995

Jargon

Verbiage justified by some as "helpful shorthand" but more often used to confuse.

Your abstract says: "Chlorothiazide induced natriuresis, kaluresis, chloruresis and bicarbonate excretion". Surely it would be better to say: "Chlorothiazide increased the excretion of sodium, potassium, chloride and bicarbonate".

George Pickering.
Chairing meeting at Royal College of Physicians, 1973

If the words are not clearly defined jargon becomes gibberish. Kahn talks of psychopaths and says he means: "Those discordant personalities which, on the causal side are characterised by quantitative peculiarities in the impulse, temperament and character strata and in their unified goal-striving activity are impaired by quantitative deviations and foreign variations".

Most of us would agree with Macdonald Critchley that this definition borders on the meaningless.

C Mawdsley. Medical pudder. *Res Medica*, 1968

Jargon intoxication

Condition that afflicts habitual jargon users, rendering them insensitive to the meaning of the words that they use.

This trial is encouraging but had insufficient power to resolve the disparity between the apparent benefit of myocardial infarction but the possible adverse effect of death.

Factfile 2/99, British Heart Foundation, 1997

This patient's impotence is causing relationship difficulties and therefore contributes to his feeling of disconnectedness.

Letter to Dr Douglas Howes, a GP in Chudleigh, Devon, from a community psychiatric nurse, 1993

Jaunty

Air adopted by doctors who think they're "good with patients" when they have to pass on disturbing news.

Diane Johnson, novelist and Professor of English at the University of California, mentions what she calls "the odd jocularity common to all gloomy professions" and cites as an example: "Well, Mrs Jones, Henry is pretty sick. We're going to run a couple of tests, have a look at that pump of his".

This translates, she says, as: "Henry is in shock. We're taking him to the radiology department to put a catheter into his aorta and inject contrast material. If he has what I think he has, he has a 42% chance of surviving".

David Woods.
Canadian Medical Association Journal, 4 October 1980

Jenner, Edward

An imposter who claimed in 1796 to be the "originator" of smallpox vaccination. The first known vaccination had been performed nearly a quarter of a century before by a Dorset farmer, Benjamin Jesty.

Sacred to the memory of Benjamin Jesty (of Downshay) who departed this life April 16, 1816 aged 79 years.
He was born in Yetminster in this County, and was an upright honest man particularly noted for having been the first Person (known) that introduced the Cow Pox by

Inoculation, and who from his great strength of mind made the Experiment from the (Cow) on his Wife and two Sons in the Year 1774.

Tombstone. St Nicholas churchyard, Worth Matravers, Isle of Purbeck, Dorset

It seems to me that Jenner must have heard what Jesty did; but there was never a mention, never an acknowledgement by him, nor is there by those who write today about the history of vaccination. Can it be a conspiracy of silence by the medical profession—starting possibly with Jenner—because the first known vaccinator was not a medical man?

Bryan Brooke. *World Medicine*, 22 September 1979

Job titles

NHS decorations awarded to **Grey Suits** in lieu of personalised number plates.

One day's crop in a single paper included a Primary Care Strategy Development Officer, a Joint Planning and Development Worker Substance Misuse, a Reprovision Consultant, a Mentoring Project Co-ordinator, a Human Resources Health Management Advisor, a Motion Analysis Scientist, numerous Clinical Studies Co-ordinators, Audit Facilitators, Operations Directors (for administrative, not surgical operations)...and Counsellors by the score.

Fritz Spiegl. *Daily Telegraph*, 12 Nov 1994

Killer bug

Virulent infection that savages newspapers. The 1994 organism, the flesh eating death bug, was no respecter of class and affected broadsheets as severely as tabloids.

After the epidemic had raged for a week, the *Sunday Times* "set the record straight" by announcing that streptococci had been the cause of bubonic plague.

Bernard Dixon. *BMJ*, 11 June 1994

1. Why did journalists ignore the textbooks?
2. Why were medical microbiologists reluctant to help them?
3. Why did some editors ignore good advice which they received from their specialist writers?
4. Why did the Public Health Laboratory Service or the Department of Health not issue a succinct briefing paper at an early stage in the whole nonsensical nightmare?

Ibid

Suggested answers:
1. Because they contain long words like "conscientious" and your modern newshound has no time to waste on consulting dictionaries.
2. Because they remembered what was published the last time they tried to enlighten the unenlightenable.
3. Because it would have spoiled a good story.
4. In the time it would have taken for a committee to be chosen and for its members to agree dates for a meeting, define an agenda, draft a statement, seek approval from the appropriate officials etc, etc, the Black Death could have swept across Europe and be coming round a second time.

Medical Monitor, 6 July, 1994

During National Flesh-devouring Deathbug from Hell Terror Week, a man arrived in the surgery with a sore throat. After light had been thrown on his tonsils and he'd been offered an explanation of his symptoms, he turned anxious eyes on me and asked: "It couldn't be that necrophilia, could it, doctor?"

Niall Robertson, Bo'ness, West Lothian.
Personal communication

Knight starvation

Affective disorder that afflicts senior doctors in their early to mid-50s. A progressive condition that deteriorates with the publication of each Honours List and, in longstanding cases, can produce serious erosion of judgment and integrity.

Some years ago, I wrote in the *BMJ* of an unnamed doctor whom I'd much admired until he achieved the knighthood he so coveted "with an act that denied the very qualities for which he'd won my respect".

103

The editor and I later received pained complaints from three people who assumed I was writing about them. I had, in fact, been writing about someone else. I still wonder what those three had been up to.

Anecdotal evidence. *Healthcare Management*, March 1993

Labels

Useful props when we feel unwell. Once named, an illness is less threatening. *See* Lohengrin effect and Nomenclature.

> Every nation has its labels for those vague symptoms that are less an illness than an inconvenience. The English attribute them to constipation or a "chill", the French to a *crise de foie*, the Germans to *Herzinsuffizienz*, and the Americans to an allergy.
>
> The symptomatology of European chauvinism.
> *Yorkshire Medicine*, Spring 1994

Laity (BMAspeak)

People who have the misfortune not to be doctors. *See* General public.

Latin

Language still used, if only in smatterings, by doctors who like to demonstrate the intellectual superiority of their calling.

> A former dean of Manchester's medical school told me of a prospective medical student who at her interview confessed, unasked and with a certain shame, that the only Latin she knew was *coitus interruptus*.
> One man's burden. *BMJ*, 13 September 1986

Laughter

Traditionally the best medicine but underrated as a surgical technique

A comely young wife, the "cynosure" of her circle, was in bed, apparently dying from swelling and inflammation of the throat, an inaccessible abscess stopping the way. She could swallow nothing; everything had been tried. Her friends were standing round the bed in misery and helplessness.

"Try her wi' a compliment", said her husband, in a not uncomic despair. She had genuine humour, as well as he; and as physiologists know, there is a sort of mental tickling which is beyond and above control, being under the reflex system, and instinctive as well as sighing. She laughed with her whole body and soul, and burst the abscess, and was well.

John Brown (1810-82). Edinburgh physician and essayist.
Horae Subsecivae: Preface.

Learned profession

(Archaic) A self regulating group of colleagues who, for the common good of humanity, share knowledge acquired through research or from experience.

(Now) Self protecting group of individuals who recognise that knowledge is a marketable commodity.

> Three representatives from our hospital recently attended a meeting sponsored by South East Thames region on developing profiles of care. The meeting was chaired by a clinician from an NHS trust where profiles of care are well developed, and the benefits to staff and patients became evident during the day. Because our hospital has just started to develop profiles of care, our audit co-ordinator later contacted the trust concerned to see whether two or three of us could visit and talk informally to some of the relevant clinicians...We were told, however, that, though this was possible, the trust would charge £300 for the information and visit.
>
> As both hospitals are NHS hospitals, trust or not, I would have thought that we could be said to have a right of access to information designed to benefit NHS patients irrespective of where they are treated. Why should we have to pay not to reinvent the wheel?
>
> P J H Venn. Letter to *BMJ*, 1 January 1994

We are surprised at P J H Venn's thinly veiled criticism of

this trust and its inaccuracy. At Central Middlesex trust we are acknowledged experts in managed care and the use of clinical protocols. Many people ask to visit the hospital to learn from our experience, and we are happy to share our skill. The demands on our time are considerable, and we have to manage this particular demand responsibly.

Martin McNicol, Graham Morgan.
Letter to *BMJ*, 26 February 1994

I thought this a selective application of market forces. How much did the Central Middlesex pay to all those patients without whose specialised experience and knowledge the trust could never have established its expertise?

Anecdotal evidence. *Medical Interface*, February 1996

Lecture

1. Process by which the notes of a teacher become the notes of a student without passing through the minds of either.
2. Academic period set aside for rest and recovery. *See* Slides, Expert.

No sleep is so deeply refreshing as that which, during lectures, Morpheus invites us so insistently to enjoy. From the standpoint of physiology, it is amazing how quickly the ravages of a short night or a long operating session can be repaired by nodding off for a few seconds at a time.

P B Medawar.
Advice to a Young Scientist, Harper and Row, 1979

In a group of people listening to a lecture, 57% are fantasising about sex, 33% are musing over a domestic incident, 7% are blank, and 3% are listening.

Medical Monitor, 12 July 1995

The late Henry Miller, one time professor of neurology and vice chancellor of the University of Newcastle upon Tyne, defined two kinds of medical lecture: those that contain slides and those that contain original thought. I've found I can manage without either, though slides do have the advantage that they introduce an element of uncertainty. This serves to keep the lecturer awake while the warm darkness that accompanies them encourages the audience to sleep, an arrangement that some would claim approaches the ideal.

A sort of vagrancy. *An Insider's Guide to the Games Doctors Play*, Gollancz, 1986

Sound advice offered in the "Press Pack" at an American scientific meeting: "Do not photograph the speakers while they are addressing the audience. Shoot them as they approach the platform".

Anecdotal evidence.
Healthcare Management, January 1995

Legacy doctors

General practitioners in private practice who achieve regular bequests from departed patients, most of whom suffered from loneliness. *See* Lucy's Disease.

Success depends on the establishment of a Regular List, an Agreed Illness, and an Agreed Prescription. *See* Harley Street doctor.

The Regular List

The foundation of legacy practice. A list of patients visited at the same time each week, each fortnight, or each month.

All had been on the Regular List for at least a year, many for 10 years, and one had had a weekly bedside consultation for the previous 22 years. Most were women whose tycoon husbands had despatched themselves to an early grave accumulating the wealth that their widows now frittered away on frivolities: expensive hairdressers, expensive boxes of chocolates, expensive flower arrangements, and expensive regular visits from an expensive private doctor.

My biggest problem was trying to discover the topics on which I was expected to converse during the hour allotted on my timetable. I soon discovered the one thing they didn't want was any form of clinical examination, other than my holding their wrist in pulse-taking mode while they told me long rambling self centred stories.

One man's burden. *BMJ*, 29 October 1983

The Agreed Illness

The foundation of the Regular List. The ideal Agreed Illness is not too incapacitating to interfere with the pleasures of a well

107

upholstered life, yet serious enough to need regular attention and to allow for occasional spectacular "attacks" that demand dramatic medical intervention and sympathetic clucking from friends.

The Agreed Illness must be specific both to patient and doctor. Patients talking to impressionable friends, must be able to say: "My liver (kidney/womb/metabolism) is unique, you know. Every doctor, and I've seen the very best, my dear, has been quite baffled by my *x* rays". But unless they can add: "Indeed they're so complicated that only dear Dr Handholder can understand them", dual specificity has not been established and patients could, after a minor tiff, take their profitable illnesses elsewhere.

One man's burden. *BMJ*, 29 October 1983

The most popular Agreed Illnesses were afflictions of the liver and alimentary tract—particularly the colon—and in setting them up, the "legacy doctor" had avoided too precise an aetiology. Most involved something that had "slipped"— womb, stomach, intervertebral disc, even an occasional rib—but there were a lot of "floating kidneys" and impressive yardages of surplus bowel. Three patients (I secretly hoped they would meet one day) told me: "Dr Handholder says I have the longest colon he's ever seen on an *x* ray". Another popular Agreed Illness was low blood pressure, which had the advantage of being the antithesis of something suffered by the common herd. Those who wished their ailments to be touched by science had settled for "sluggish metabolism" or "disturbed biochemistry".

Ibid

The Agreed Prescription
The only antidote to the Agreed Illness.

This was always a mixture of at least six innocuous items; any fewer would have been unimposing when written on the prescription and any active ingredient might produce an unpleasant physiological effect. The mixture also had to have an unpleasant taste. Regular Visits had a masochistic streak. They were born to suffer from the Agreed Illness and relief came only out of tribulation.

The other standard treatment was the Agreed Injection, usually of cytamen. Its pink colour helped it home in vigorously on the placebo receptors. I suspected an Agreed

Injection had converted many a patient from an occasional to a Regular Visit because injections never came singly but in courses, no course had a predetermined length, and no course could be effective without an unspecified number of reinforcing courses.

> One man's burden. *BMJ*, 29 October 1983

Levity

A cathartic activity in which doctors who wish to succeed have to overindulge when they are students and underindulge once they are registered. *See* Qualification.

> He has risen by his gravity and I have been sunk by my levity.
> Sydney Smith (of his brother).
> Quoted in *Medical Interface*, December 1995

Life enhancing services

Self enhancing title recently assumed by local authority health services.

> In Tameside Metropolitan Borough, clinical psychology is offered by a department called Life Enhancing Services. All very worthy but the same title could be used by any pub, restaurant, cinema, or other place of entertainment of good or ill repute—provided, of course, it had the same air of self importance and lack of self consciousness as Tameside Metropolitan Borough.
> *Audiomonitor*, September 1995

Life threatening

Fashionable phrase that, despite its ambiguity, has become a top of the market euphemism. The *Sun*'s "killer Bug" is the *Daily Telegraph*'s "dangerous illness" and the *BMJ*'s "life threatening disease".

Andrew Brooke, a Gloucester GP, noticed that one of the

criteria for referral to a workshop at the Gloucestershire Royal Hospital devoted to "Understanding Grief" was that the death must have occurred as a result of a life threatening illness. As opposed, asks Dr Brooke, to illnesses that threaten death?

Medical Monitor, 5 April 1997

Much favoured by people who seek to impress with the sound rather than the meaning of what they say. *See* Trustspeak, BMAspeak.

Since Christmas, we have had to postpone all but the most life threatening surgery.

Memo from Royal Berkshire and Battle Hospitals to local GPs, February 1997

Linguistic autoimmunity

Rare syntactical condition in which words become allergic to their own meaning.

"I'm very worried about our marriage", said an anxious husband. "I'm afraid that if my wife's agoraphobia gets any worse she is going to walk out".
Peter Moore, Torquay GP. *Medical Monitor*, 28 April 1993

I'd give my right arm to be able to play the guitar.
Ambulance driver at Royal Surrey Hospital, January 1997

Literalism

An interpretative disorder first described by Denis Norden. A congenital inability to interpret words other than literally.

On being confronted with the headline PUBLIC BORROWING DOWN, my instinctive response was "What a strange thing for members of the public to be borrowing. Just shows how many people must be stuffing their own duvets".

And when I turned to the Arts Page and found a story headed HOCKNEY DRAWS LARGE CROWDS, the immediate thought was, "Well, I suppose it must make a change from drawing swimming pools"...
Denis Norden. *You Have my Word*, Mandarin, 1989

Dr Peter Kersey, a Plymouth dermatologist can't understand why are were so many signs in his hospital indicating "Disabled Toilet" when people need to be directed to the working ones.

> Anecdotal evidence. *Medical Interface*, July 1996

Julian Churcher, a South West London GP, spotted this entry on a temporary resident form (FP19) completed by a French visitor:

> Name of Doctor at home: DOCTEUR.
> *Medical Monitor*, 15 January 1993

Dr A P Harrison of Keighley suffers deprivation every time he visits a department store in Cardiff where a notice in the cafe reads: "'All our tea is served in China". Not much use, says Dr Harrison, to a person dying of thirst in South Wales.

> Anecdotal evidence. *Medical Interface*, January 1996

Literature, The

Presumptuous title given to gobbets of ill-written prose published in the guise of **scientific papers.**

> As things are, too much of what passes for the scientific literature is not literature at all but a way of stringing code words together in such a way that the perpetrators can enjoy the warm glow of knowing that a piece of research has been written up and given a prominent place on the library shelves throughout the world....The immediate interests of readers that they should be able to read and understand are given only scant attention.
> John Maddox, editor, Nature.
> In: *Communicating Science: A Handbook*, Longman, 1991

Little prick

Phrase used by patronising doctors to describe an injection that is not too painful, as in "You'll just feel a little prick". Also a description of the sort of person who uses the phrase.

Local medical society

Group of apathetic doctors nagged by hyperactive secretary whose job is to invite an **expert** and then try desperately to assemble an audience.

> Secretaries usually greet you at the station or airport and drive you to the appointed place. They then park you in a room with a large mug of coffee while they keep popping anxiously next door to see if anyone has turned up. Their conversation consists entirely of hints that the audience is likely to be slim. They talk of the atrocious weather, the football on television, the local concert being given that evening by James Galway, John Denver or the Halle Orchestra, the Annual Ball that most of their members attended the previous night.
>
> A sort of vagrancy. *An Insider's Guide to the Games Doctors Play*, Gollancz, 1986

> An essential attribute for such a person is indomitable optimism. Beryl Bainbridge has described how a fellow author, invited to address a meeting, found himself, one hour after the meeting was due to start, in a hall that contained only the chairman, the caretaker, and himself.
>
> "Shall we pack it in?" asked the author.
>
> "Not yet", said the chairman. "Best wait for stragglers".
>
> *Ibid*

Lohengrin effect

Loss of power effected by the giving of a name. A traditional therapeutic tool. *See* Labels.

> Lohengrin arrives on a swan just in time to save Elsa. He becomes her hero and promises to marry her as long as she doesn't ask him his name. Yet, hardly has the last bar of the wedding march faded when Elsa, displaying the sort of boneheadedness without which there would be no legends and precious few operas, asks the forbidden question and Lohengrin catches the next swan back up the Scheldt.
>
> This theme of people losing their power once they are named recurs in fables from Rumpelstiltskin through *Turandot* to *Last Tango in Paris*. It also recurs regularly in medicine.

"Is this throat of mine serious?" asks the patient.
"No", says the doctor. "Just pharyngitis".
"Good", says the patient. The evil has lost its power. It has a name. That's even more reassuring than a treatment and certainly has fewer side effects.
The toxic effect of language on medicine. *Journal of the Royal College of Physicians*, November/December 1995

I admit shamefully that I occasionally used the Lohengrin effect in general practice when a patient showed me a prescription or thrust a handful of tablets under my nose and asked: "Is this a drug, doctor?"
If I wanted them to take the tablets I said "No"; if I thought they'd be better of without them, I said "Yes".

Ibid

Reverse Lohengrin effect
In this variation the doctor transfers the labels, and power, to the patients.

I spent an uneasy fortnight as a locum in a practice where mothers of children with bellyache were told that their child had "acidosis" and patients with indeterminate minor symptoms were told they had "low blood pressure". These syndromes shared two characteristics: the sufferers were all private patients and their conditions needed regular scientific attention from their GP. Mothers had to consult him about the changes they needed to make in their children's diets "to readjust the acidity of the system". Patients with "low blood pressure" had to have prophylactic injections of Vitamin B12 to ward off the diverse symptoms their condition seemed to produce.
The treatments brought rich rewards, and not just to the doctor. The mothers found a new obsessional purpose in their lives as they strove to balance their children's diets, the children had a ready made excuse with which to remove themselves from any unpleasing circumstance, and the vitamin injections, because of their pink colour, homed in vigorously on the placebo receptors. When I suggested alternative labels, or hinted that maybe no label was needed, the patients withdrew their patronage and accommodated their symptoms until my master's return.
The Lohengrin game. *An Insider's Guide to the Games Doctors Play*, Gollancz, 1986

113

Loud and clear (BMAspeak)

How our message must go out.

Lucre, filthy, disinterest in

Traditional ingredient of the bedside manner

> A physician should take his fee without letting his left hand know what his right hand is doing; it should be taken without a thought, without a look, without a move of the facial muscles; the true physician should hardly be aware that the last friendly grasp of the hand had been made more precious by the touch of gold.
>
> Anthony Trollope. *Doctor Thorne*, 1858

Lucy's disease

An affliction of proud, lonely persons. Eponym suggested by Richard Asher.

> She dwelt among the untrodden ways
> Beside the springs of Dove,
> A maid whom there were none to praise
> And very few to love.
>
> William Wordsworth. *Lucy*

To lonely people a medical consultation may represent an event of great importance. It supplies that need to be noticed that exists in all human beings. A child cries: "Look at my sand castle!" A lonely old person cries: "Look at my stomach". The child says: "I got two goals this afternoon!" The lonely old person says: "I got two giddy turns this afternoon".

I have heard, from more than one practitioner, of elderly people who have a weekly or fortnightly consultation of this kind. A visit from the doctor allows them the illusion of seeking medical advice rather than companionship. A patient may be too proud to complain of loneliness, but there is no loss of pride in complaining of symptoms.

Lonely people miss not only companionship but also the advice and criticism that go with it. Under the guise of seeking advice about health, a lonely lady may be seeking advice about family affairs. Ostensibly she is asking for

advice about her bad heart, but *au fond* she seeks advice about her bad nephew.
Richard Asher.

Richard Asher Talking Sense, Pitman Medical, 1972

Lump Index

A model for predicting which patients may be susceptible to **counselling**.

> The Index, devised over dinner with encouragement from Henry Miller, is best explained by describing cases at each end of the scale.
>
> A cultured man with a slight blemish on the back of his hand may enjoy a session with a doctor who explores his social background, disentangles the psychodynamics of anxiety and conflict in his work and family, and whose conversation has the vision of a Renaissance man.
>
> An equally cultured man whose lump is the size of a football, red and angry-looking, with sinuous blood vessels throbbing across its surface, might grow fractious as the Renaissance doctor gently explored the premarital relationship that existed between his grandparents, might even look over the doctor's shoulder seeking a gruff butcher with a sharp knife.
>
> *Medical Monitor*, 13 July 1990

Mace

Gilded reproduction of outdated weapon of war much favoured by medical institutions. Rarely put to useful purpose, though Michael Heseltine once swung the House of Commons mace around his head and burned off excess cathecholamines when he might otherwise have done something dangerous, like sitting down and thinking.

> Anthony Clare once told me that, when the college of psychiatrists was being founded, the longest and most heated discussion was over whether this new, exciting, and different college should have a mace. In the end, he said, the

pro-macers won because the anti-macers could not rebut the argument that "a mace will help to open doors".
One man's burden. *BMJ*, 20 July 1985

Major Breakthrough (Hackspeak)

Cashiered officer who makes regular appearances in the tabloids.

One of my patients hadn't spoken for 20 years until she started getting the injections. An excited sister summoned me to the bedside.
"What did she say, sister?"
She said: "Arseholes to you, doctor".
"Anything else?"
"No, nothing. But it's a major breakthrough".
Norman Imlah. Speaking at press conference. In: *World Medicine*, 10 March 1970

Malaproposis

Form of dysphasia that enables patients to demonstrate to their doctors that the *mot juste* is not always the *mot évidente*.

One Tottenham family looked after by John Nixon is suing the council because of its failure to rehouse them. Recently, when invited to inspect the children's bedroom yet again, he was told: "Just look at all that compensation on the walls".
Medical Monitor, 16 October 1996

When a patient at Paul Walton's surgery in Sacriston asked for "Flymogel" sachets the doctor feared the poor man's lawn mower had seized up and needed a catharsis.
Medical Monitor, 23 August 1995

An elderly lady patient telephoned me today to complain about side effects of the new tablets the hospital had given her...Insubordinate Mononitrate.
David Davies, Haverfordwest, Pembrokeshire.
Personal communication

I've had a vivacious cyst removed and now need some Ferocious Sulphate for my blood.
Paul Dewhirst, Normanton, West Yorkshire.
Personal communication

Brian Hamilton knew that summer had arrived in Stanstead when an 80 year old lady asked him to prescribe her old treatment, "phenobarbecue tablets".

Monitor Weekly, 2 June 1994

When Charles Simenoff of Crumpsall was asked by a patient suffering from acid reflux if it would help if she had a Bavarian Meal, Dr Simenoff wasn't sure that chocolate cake was quite the ticket.

Ibid

In Manchester Dr Stanley Goodman was disconcerted when a man asked for a prescription for Dulux suppositories. No doubt he was seeking a high gloss finish.

Monitor Weekly, 14 September 1994

I could name a few patients who would match the description that a surgeon used when he wrote to Dr A M McEwen of Buckhurst Hill. "Your patient is a keen player in her local bowels team".

Medical Monitor, 9 August 1995

Masturbation

A disease that so ravaged the flower of English youth in the 19th and early 20th centuries that leaders of men had to issue stern explicit advice.

The frame is stunted and weak, the muscles under-developed, the eye is sunken and heavy, the complexion is sallow, pasty, or covered with spots of acne, the hands are damp and cold, and the skin moist. The boy shuns the society of others, creeps about alone, joins with repugnance in the amusements of his schoolfellows. He cannot look anyone in the face, and becomes careless in dress and uncleanly in person. His intellect has become sluggish and enfeebled, and if his evil habits are persisted in, he may end in becoming a drivelling idiot or a peevish valetudinarian.
Dr William Acton. *The Function and Disorders of the Reproductive Organs in Childhood, Youth, Adult Age, and Advanced Life, Considered in their Physiological, Social and Moral Relations,* 1857

Apathy, loss of memory, abeyancy of concentrative power

and manifestation of mind generally, combined with loss of self reliance, and indisposition for or impulsiveness of action, irritability of temper, and incoherence of language, are the most characteristic mental phenomena of chronic dementia resulting from masturbation.

Ibid

The printer, Horace Cox, refused to print the first edition of Baden-Powell's *Scouting for Boys* in 1908 until some "far too explicit" advice was removed, including the wholesome advice offered to boys who felt the urge coming on—"Just wash your parts in cold water and cool them down".

The version Cox eventually printed was so enigmatic that many a scout must have wondered what exactly was the dangerous activity against which he was being warned. "This 'beastliness' is not a man's vice; men have nothing but contempt for a fellow who gives way to it".

Anecdotal evidence.
Healthcare Management, October 1993

Management

The art of disposing of difficult clinical or administrative problems by using three "core" techniques:
- Delegation of responsibility
- Appropriation of credit
- Shifting of blame.

Marginalised

Trustspeak for "ignored". Over the past decade Britain has lead the way in extending the vocabulary of deprivation.

Christine Tyrie, a consultant psychiatrist in Carlisle, described how those struggling to cope with non-existent "care in the community" could no longer refer to "unmet needs". They were dealing instead with "preferred option shortfall".

Anecdotal evidence.
Healthcare Management, November 1994

Market system

Administrative strategy believed to be the only way to bring efficiency to health services—but only by people who are aged under 60 or have lost their memory. *See* Internal market.

> The health services during the interwar period...contained many of the elements of the market system towards which there is now a reversion. The voluntary hospitals proved unable to meet the demands of medical modernisation. In response to their precarious situation, the leaders of the voluntary hospitals recognised that the future hospital services would depend on public subsidy and differ in their method of management and organisation. Experience had demonstrated that the market system was a failure.
>
> Charles Webster, Senior Research Fellow,
> All Souls. *Lecture to Royal College of Physicians*,
> 18 July 1995

> The remarkable improvements in health care brought about under the planned system were achieved by methods contrary to market principles and which rejected the purchaser/provider split. Even according to narrow criteria of efficiency gains, the achievements of the early NHS were of an altogether higher order than anything claimed for the current wave of experimentation with market systems. The forms of administration and management introduced by Bevan were not an irresponsible and wasteful experiment in socialism, but the logical conclusion of an evolutionary development which had been underway for more than a decade. It is therefore the early NHS, not the chimeras of the marketeers, which represents the realisation of Britain's native genius in the field of health care.
>
> *Ibid*

Medical advice column

Traditional outlet for doctors who enjoy patronising non-doctors. *Private Eye*'s "A doctor writes..." draws on a long tradition.

> A boil is of no practical value. It is said that everything has its use, but this certainly does not apply to boils. They are of no use; and few people consider them ornamental. They do

not improve your personal appearance, and they do not add to your comfort.

We are told, on good authority, that in many cases they must be looked upon as salutary, as being the means adopted by Nature to rid the system of morbid matters that irritate the constitution. This may be, but a boil is a violent remedy. Most people, if they had the choice, would prefer a less energetic means of having the system cleared out. Scientific doctors usually call them furunculi, but even then they are rather painful.

Physicians and Surgeons of the Principal London Hospitals.
The Family Physician, 1883

Medical Curriculum, revising the

Traditional game played by **educationalists** to well established rules.

- Virtually anything that is new will be popular at the time of its introduction and for a few years thereafter because the medical course is so dull
- At least 75% of innovations will have a half life of less than five years
- Long range experiments to test the validity or relevance of educational change are doomed to fail because patterns of practice, of demand, and of need will also have changed by the time evaluation is made
- Policy statements about the curriculum are either so vague as to be empty or so jargon-ridden as to be incomprehensible
- "Goals", "objectives", and "problems" are the catch words of ill formulated theory rather than the precise components of intelligent dialogue. "Orientation" should be dropped from the technical vocabulary
- Those persons who talk about teaching "principles" rarely (if ever) know what they mean
- Multidisciplinary laboratories/courses/seminars etc, are fine as long as there is one for each discipline
- The inevitable outcome of having a curriculum committee is a loss of real interest in medical education, but if one does not exist it should be invented to keep busy those who want change.

Hugh Dudley. *World Medicine*, 30 November 1977

Medical Establishment

Loose knit group of powerful doctors who have within their gift not just the best jobs but all the appurtenances that distinguish the gentlemen from the players.

> For the academically inclined, they can gain access to research funds, consultancies to international agencies, and regular invitations to symposia in places like Florence, Tokyo, San Francisco, or Barbados. For those keen to succeed in private practice, they can arrange membership of dining clubs and appearances at postgraduate meetings which get a chap's name known within the trade. And for those with a taste for pomp, they give regular leg-ups on the beanstalk that has its roots in administrative and political committees and grows into the cloudborne land of gold chains, mutual votes of thanks, and the reassuring touch of sword on shoulder.
>
> Like all good Establishments, the system that distributes this patronage is not an organised network with a Mr Big skulking at its centre but an ill-defined scatter of well-meaning fellows, dropping a word here, a hint there, and earning each other's co-operation by lending support here, withdrawing it there. Indeed some are unaware of the power that they wield and take a naive delight in the success that seems to smile upon the decent young fellows they know.
>
> The patronage game. *An Insider's Guide to the Games Doctors Play*, Gollancz, 1986

Medical history, taking an interest in

Displacement activity disguised as study. Appeals to middle aged doctors who have grown bored with the routine of clinical practice.

Medical sesquipedalianism

A love not just of long words but of long sentences.

> With regard to the aetiology of his intellect and behaviour immaturity, secondary to the failure of the normal ontoge-

netic unfolding of the neocortical portions of the cerebral cortex, this is probably a genetically determined cause.

Medical report quoted in *Journal of the American Medical Association*, 20 January 1969, by Edmund J Simpson who translates it: "This boy's mental retardation is congenital"

Medicine and the Media

Popular subject for meetings of **local medical societies** when committee discovers that scientific subjects draw small audiences.

A couple of posh journalists are invited and the rubric is depressingly predictable: an hour or two of polite exchange of grudge and prejudice topped off with a moment of consensual high mindedness. Then the hacks rejoin the world of headlines like *Pooftahs in the Pulpit* and the doctors with a mission to explain go home to scold their juniors for allowing patients to see what's written in their notes.

The trouble is that Medicine and Media are blanket words and, like other blankets, cover multifarious activities. When used in tandem they describe a territory so broad it invites folk to range across it, scavenge in selected areas, then shape their scavengings to fit any theory they wish to purvey.

The medical condition. *The Listener*, 12 May 1988

Mediocrity

Infection difficult to eradicate from medical institutions. Inevitable product of patronage. Luckily for us all it is usually a self limiting condition.

Mediocre persons, with nothing to defend but their unmerited authority, use patronage to repel all intrusion by imagination, initiative or enterprise and may dominate a hospital for as long as 12 years.

Then they are usually overthrown because, thank God, the patronage system carries within it the seeds of its own subversion. Doctors who actually practise medicine, as opposed to those who play political games, really do enjoy their work and one of their rewards is some insight into the strange ways in which folk behave—including the folk they have to work with. Given the provocation, they will divert their attention temporarily from their true love and make radical changes in their institutions.

> One man's burden. *BMJ*, 3 August 1985

Methodology

Noun added as seasoning to oatmeal prose to give it a "scientific" flavour. *See* Decorated Municipal Gothic.

> Dr J N Blau of the National Hospital, Queen Square, asks those who use the word: "Have you ever taken your children to the zoology in Regent's Park?"
>
> Anecdotal evidence. *Medical Interface*, September 1996

Miracle

Spontaneous remission of illness. A common occurrence. Earns title "miracle" only if it follows unorthodox treatment or the patient needs to deify the doctor.

> Life itself is too great a miracle for us to make so much fuss about potty little reversals of what we pompously assume to be the natural order.
>
> Robertson Davies. *Fifth Business*, Penguin, 1970

Mission Statements

Pious utterances that Trusts print beneath the expensively commissioned logo on their notepaper.

> Working together for health
> *Aylesbury Vale Community Health Care Trust*

> Your partner for Health
> *Camden and Islington Community Health Services NHS Trust*

> Caring for one & all
> *Royal Cornwall Hospitals Trust*

Putting Patients First
Green Park Healthcare Trust

Improving the health of the nation
Department of Health

"Who dreams them up? They are as right-minded and meaningless as an 18th century epitaph without any of the elegance".
Rennick Baxter. *Medical Interface*, January 1996

During one coccyx-numbing meeting Rennick Baxter looked down at the notepad placed before him and saw he had doodled under the Trust logo: "Creating Tomorrow's Problems Today".
Anecdotal evidence. *Medical Interface*, January 1996

Similar pieties, in expanded form, can be found at entrances to wards and clinics.

The philosophy of care in this ward aims to deliver holistic individualised family centred care meeting the needs of both the hospitalised child and their [sic] families.
Notice outside a Sheffield paediatric ward.

Who are they aimed at? We patients, burdened with pains and aches, and even more frightening intimations of mortality, have little intellectual space left in which to ponder insubstantialities like "philosophies of care".

If, as most of us believe, the doctors and nurses are trying to do their best for us, we'd prefer to read that message in their actions than in ill-constructed statements on the wall. And if they start telling us too loudly just how clever they are we may begin to wonder if they feel as insecure as we do.

I suspect the exercise is designed to impress any passing manager who's recently been on a Ongoing Communications course and whose space between the ears is so stuffed with Business Plans, Protocols, and Paradigms it has become a nous-free area.
Anecdotal evidence. *Medical Interface*, May 1996

Model

Word stolen from the world of research, where it has a specific meaning, and used to add "scientific" weight to woolly statements.

The medical model does not offer the right route of access to the understanding of these patients' problems.
Paper presented at Symposium on Social Psychiatry, 1989

The model we need is a remodel of the model that has led to this catastrophic shortfall.
Speaker at emergency meeting of West Surrey Health Authority, April 1997

Modesty

Becoming quality still found in some patients.

> Mom used to insist that Aunt Edie wasn't a wicked person, just a frightened one. So frightened, apparently, that whenever she visited her gynecologist, she took a special bag with her to wear on her head during cervical examinations.
> Armistead Maupin. *Maybe the Moon*, Black Swan, 1992

Moment in time
See End of day.

Mortality

1. The only incurable disease. Too often regarded by doctors as an enemy to be fought on every front rather than an awkward ally who has occasionally to be appeased.
2. A concept that confuses journalists.

> Teetotallers run a greater risk of dying than drinkers who consume in moderation, say researchers.
> Press release. *Edinburgh Science Festival*, 1993

Ms Spell

Ubiquitous medical secretary who strives to enhance her employer's messages.

In Kingsthorpe, Dr J M Griffin received a slip of paper—indeed a Freudian slip of paper—inviting him to a discussion of the new complaints procedure which "comes into farce on April 1".

And in Luton, a consultant offered Margaret Thomson a helpful piece of advice about a patient who was experiencing dyspareunia. "They should also consider using lubricants to rejuice the resistance when Mr X penetrates his wife".

Medical Monitor, 15 May 1996

Not all misprints endow as felicitous a meaning as that in a sentence addressed to Dr A G Martynoga in Dalkeith. "By the time of admission, he had improved 'about 50%' and was talking to the toilet".

Medical Monitor, 8 January 1993

Mark Davis of Sidcup received this specialist report on a patient with persistent hyperacidity: "His reflux symptoms were kept under control with anti-secretary therapy"—an anti-dyspeptic measure that I suspect is underused.

Medical Monitor, 2 October 1996

Muddling through

Managerial philosophy that, despite expensive attempts to find alternatives, has enabled the NHS to survive—just.

I can't remember a time when the NHS didn't face some sort of "crisis": a dispute over levels of pay between government and nurses or government and doctors, a shortage of beds in certain specialities, long waiting lists for elective surgery and so on. Yet despite regular warnings that the system was in danger of imminent collapse it somehow managed to survive for over 40 years thanks to the British tradition of "muddling through" and because the service was still imbued with the altruism with which it had been launched.

The Pharos, Winter 1996

The NHS would long since have collapsed if it were not for the stalwart efforts of the majority who believe in it and work their backsides off to keep it going.

Neil Watson. Letter, *BMJ*, 18 January 1997

I may hate administration, get bored crazy by committees,

believe that contracts are based more on dogma than on the real world, find some patients and colleagues a pain in the neck—but I still love my job. The more I put in the more I get out of it.

William Notcutt. *BMA News Review*, 2 August 1995

No doubt times are bad; history suggests that perhaps they always were bad, for the great majority of people. The future of the health service depends on our recovering cheerfulness and dedication; the future of our own profession depends on a shared idealism.

Sir Douglas Black. The paradox of medical care. *Journal of the Royal College of Physicians of London*, 2 April 1979

Murphy

Apocryphal law maker. Laws attributed to him by doctors include:

It is easier to get into something than to get out of it.
Whatever you have to do, you have to do something else first.
Nothing is impossible to those who don't have to do it themselves.
No good deed goes unpunished.
Leak-proof seals will.
Interchangeable parts won't.

Myeloencephalitis (ME)

Illness characterised by an overwhelming sense of lassitude that drains sufferers of energy to do anything except engage in vigorous argument with anyone who suggests their illness has a psychological component.

Myxmetaphorosis

Hyperactivity of the "creative communications" centre. Most often induced by overexposure to management courses but can affect medical authors with literary aspirations.

As the concept of wrongful life swims upon the precarious seas of judicial reasoning, one wonders whether it will serve forth a veritable Pandora's box of litigation to become a fish bone in the throat of obstetric practice.

John Gardner. Trends in medico-legal aspects of contraception, *Clinics in Obstetrics and Gynecology: Contraception, Saunders, April 1979*

Since then he has served as a bipartisan consultant to several governments, furthering his reputation as a creative egg cracker in medicopolitical cake baking. And the cake of long waiting lists and spiralling costs needs the cracking of an emu sized egg...

Simon Chapman. *BMJ*, 12 November 1994

A memo sent to David McKinlay's medical audit group exhorted it to promote a conference with the stirring cry: "Please cascade this flyer through your network".

Audiomonitor, September 1996

Name badges

1. Labels issued to hospital staff to prevent them from stealing one another's white coats.
2. Labels issued at medical school **reunions**. (Of little value. At early reunions people are still recognisable derivatives of what they once were. At later meetings when physical change *does* impede identification, few can read the labels without bending embarrassingly close.)

Natural

Not man made and therefore wholesome. Highly effective marketing "concept" in the 1980s and '90s.

As a doctor I don't see Nature as a benevolent matriarch. My profession spends a lot of time trying to insulate human beings from the effects of natural catastrophes or trying to repair bodies and minds that have been visited by an often malevolent Mother Nature. Indeed medicine's job is to protect people from the ravages of our often hostile natural environment and, when protection fails, to try and repair the damage...The law still recognises that most people die of natural causes.

How to Succeed in Business Without Sacrificing your Health, 1988

Nature has no bias and can be seen at work as clearly, and as inexorably, in the spread of an epidemic as in the birth of a healthy baby.

Looking sideways. *Medical Monitor*, 25 January 1991

The principal task of civilisation, its actual *raison d'être* is to defend us against nature.

Sigmund Freud. Quoted in: *A Gentleman Publisher's Commonplace Book*, John Murray, 1996

Natural childbirth

Doctor-free parturition. Phrase coined in the 1920s and '30s by campaigners who wanted to free women from the need for analgesia during labour. Since annexed by groups promoting any unusual way of conducting childbirth.

And what could be more natural than a woman giving birth while naked, supported by a hairy French doctor singing *La Marseillaise*, and dropping the baby into a plastic paddling pool full of dirty, tepid salt water?

Russell Ash. *The Cynic's Dictionary*, Corgi, 1983

Negativism

A not uncommon professional quirk that makes it not unusual for medical writers not to accentuate the positive.

The fact that there is no evidence to believe that they are due to tuberculosis or mental illness would not necessarily lead me to conclude that they are not due to these things, but it would lead me to conclude that there was no reason to believe that these causes were responsible for the pain and disability in his back.

Orthopaedic report quoted by Edmund J Simpson. *Verba sesquipedalia. Journal of the American Medical Association*, 20 January 1969

Newsflash

Sparks that fly when the news desk reaches for the medical dictionary.

Minister rapped over organs

New Scientist, 1 January 1977

The injury is not, as has been widely reported, a groin injury. He is suffering from symphysis pubis.

Sunday Times, 1978

KIRWAN RECOVERS. National Organiser Lawrence Kirwan is now recuperating from an operation for hernia and hopes to be back in harness in early November

The Journalist. Official organ of the National Union of Journalists, 10 November 1976

A psychiatrist for the defendant said that he was suffering from a psychiatric condition known as ambivalence.

Oxford Times, May 1996

NHS Statistics

Public relations data seasonally adjusted to meet the needs of the Department of Health. *See* Waiting lists, Spin doctor.

The "indicators of success" quoted by government politicians today bear a strong similarity to those published shortly before the 1992 general election. They were unconvincing then, and time has not improved them.

The statistics are far too limited to enable a proper assessment of the impact of changes in the NHS, and even the statistics provided do not support the interpretations government politicians place on them. NHS statistics, like the NHS itself, are still not safe in politicians' hands.

Improvements are needed in the collection and publication of statistics.

NHS "indicators of success": What do they tell us?

BMJ, 28 January 1995

The explanation given for the mix up over figures released last week on NHS spending has left statisticians puzzled and confused. On 30 January the Office for National Statistics withdrew from sale the latest edition of *Social Trends* after claiming that a chart which showed that government spending on the NHS had fallen by £1bn over three years in real terms was a mistake. The figures ran contrary to ministers repeated declarations that NHS spending under the Conservative government has increased year on year.

Within 24 hours of the "error" having been spotted, the Office for National Statistics issued an amended version of the chart showing that government spending has risen consistently.

Zosia Kmietowicz. Confusion reigns over official health statistics. *BMJ*, 8 February 1997

Niche

New NHS marketing title for a person previously known as a "customer" or, back in the Dark Ages, a "patient".

Dr Mark Baker, the Bradford Hospital Trust's chief executive, told a conference of health service managers that he wants clinical practice to become a "high value-added niche service, in which every patient is a niche", a concept which I'm sure few GPs will question—or even understand.

Medical Monitor, 1 May 1992

Nightfall

Mystical fading of the light that ushers in the hours of medical eccentricity.

Dr Ford Simpson of Hawick was disturbed in the early hours by a 'phone call from the local Community Care

Alarm System that responds to signals from panic buttons supplied to elderly people. He was told that a patient had pressed her alarm button but was so distressed she could only wheeze her message over the intercom. Dr Simpson quickly attended the scene and found the patient comfortably asleep in her bed. Her large dog had climbed alongside her and had pressed the panic button with his nose.

Medical Monitor, 6 November 1992

One evening when Harry was working as a casualty officer at St Luke's Hospital in Bradford, a nurse entered his domain in a fair old panic. A disturbed elderly lady had vanished from her ward and could be found nowhere in the hospital. Harry, being a kindly soul, offered to get out his car and go and look for the absconder.

He'd travelled barely half a mile when he spotted his quarry wandering along the pavement in her nightdress. Though she was highly confused, he managed to get her into the passenger seat and drove her back to the hospital where he left her locked in the car while he went to find her keepers. As he re-entered the hospital the nurse rushed up to him, thanked him for his kindness, and explained there was no need to panic because they'd found the missing woman on another ward.

Were this an apocryphal story that is where it would end. In real life, Harry and his fellow casualty officer were unable to identify the woman and were frightened to admit her because their surgeon boss had given them strict orders not to block his beds with elderly people. Eventually at 3 am, after protracted negotiations, they managed to get her admitted to a Salvation Army hostel.

The following morning the leader of Bradford City Council rang St Luke's demanding the names of the doctors who had abducted his aunt when she went out for a breath of fresh air.

Monitor Weekly, 1 December 1993

Nomenclature

Cardinal source of doctors' power. Knowing the name of a thing gives power to those who know it. *See* Labels and Lohengrin effect.

In the New Testament the words "name" and "power" are synonymous. The power to name things, to classify acts and actors, is the greatest power in the world.

Thomas Szasz. Quoted in Open Day Lecture,
Royal College of Physicians, 6 July 1995

"What is this strange skin condition with red rings which expand from the centre in widening circles?"

"That", says the dermatologist, "is erythema annular centrifugum".

He has spoken the words of power, and the dignity of the profession has been upheld.

Richard Asher. *Richard Asher Talking Sense*,
Pitman Medical, 1972

Nor bring, to see me cease to live,
Some doctor full of phrase and fame,
To shake his sapient head and give
The ill he cannot cure a name.

Matthew Arnold. *A Wish*, 1867

Nominal aphasia

One of life's milestones. Prodromal stage of serious bewilderment.

There will come a time when you will walk into a crowded room, all the faces will be familiar, and the only name you will remember will be Alzheimer's.

Robin Steel, Worcester GP. *Personal communication*

Since the departure of Mrs Thatcher the "Prime Minister" question has become a less specific test for identifying the Seriously Bewildered.

I often come across fairly lucid people who can't name John Major. The last old boy I asked to name the Prime Minister said "Smith". I said: "Actually, it's Major". Without batting an eyelid he shot back: "Oh yes, of course. Major Smith".

Peter Burke, Oxford GP.
Medical Monitor, 15 November 1995

First you forget names, then you forget faces. Next you forget to pull your zipper up and finally you forget to pull it down.

George Burns.
Quoted in *Medical Monitor*, 19 February 1997

Nominal dysphasia

Speech defect that afflicts otherwise healthy persons when they encounter someone whose name is difficult to pronounce.

> At a recent meeting I heard Professor John Guillebaud referred to under three different sounding names. Two of them were used by the same speaker so the uninitiated probably assumed that each reference was to a different person.
>
> *Medical Monitor*, 17 November 1993

> When the actress Deborah Kerr moved from Britain to Hollywood she was irritated by people who regularly mispronounced her name as "Miss Cur" rather than "Miss Car". Such was her irritation that she asked the studio to make sure that the man who summoned the stars' limousines after her next premiere would be briefed to pronounce her name properly.
>
> The studio did its stuff and after the performance the announcer, who'd been concentrating all evening on getting the pronunciation right, called over the loudspeakers for Miss Carr's car. Lulled by this success, his brain slipped into automatic drive and his next call amplified down Hollywood Boulevard was for "Mr Hitchcar's cock".
>
> *Ibid*

Nominal hypertrophy

Underpublicised feature of practising medicine in a multiethnic society

> An interesting problem arose this afternoon in that the Abdul Malik who came to the clinic was the father of the Abdul Malik whom you referred. In contrast, the notes brought from Records were for the Abdul Malik who is the son of Abdul Malik whom you referred.
>
> Various Abdul Maliks were sent round to the Record office to make an appointment for the correct Abdul Malik who will attend with Abdul Malik, an interpreter, at an

appropriate clinic. Malik seems to be a surname similar to Smith.

Medical Monitor, 15 November 1995

The patient was identified as Muhammad Rahman Mubarraq bin Ali Bellamchi. He said he was an artist and had come to this country to make a name for himself.

Looking sideways. Medical Monitor, 8 March 1991

Normal

Unremarkable and of no interest to doctors.

Note taking

The habit of doodling while the patient talks. Wise doctors discover that if they write too much, they miss most of what is being said and all of what is being implied. For the sake of appearances they may jot reminders to themselves to call at the bank or to collect something from the cleaners.

> Even when relevant, the notes are often uninformative. I once worked for a psychiatrist who after a two hour, probing, indepth, etc, interview with a patient, wrote: "Jolly little woman".
> Health warning: doctors' notes are bad for the ego.
> Times, 4 September 1981

Doctors who specialise in diseases of the rich make extensive notes to enable them to pick up the conversation where they last laid it down—notes like "handicap 18" or "daughter starts next term at Benenden" or "shrub outside bedroom window is Acer talmatum dissectum atropurpureum".

One man's burden. BMJ, 10 November 1984

Abbreviations can cause problems. I never dared explain to a patient who saw me scrawl KUTA on her notes that I'd decided she had grown too dependent on me and that at our next meeting I would try to deliver a metaphorical kick up the usual place in an effort to terminate our ongoing relationship.

One man's burden. BMJ, 15 March 1986

135

Nouns

Words that doctors use instead of verbs and adjectives.

> I have consented his mother for the operation.
> *Surgeon writing to Dr Steven R Stern of Staplecross*, 1994

> Subsequently, he was casted and six weeks thereafter was ambulated with crutches.
> Orthopaedic report quoted by Edmund J Simpson, Verba sesquipedalia. *Journal of the American Medical Association*, 20 January 1969

> A skilful linguist but habitual liar once told me of a single word in German standing for "the window of the man who issued tickets at reduced prices for admission on Sundays to the zoo". This is untrue, of course, but it illustrates the principle, and if I myself have not read about "vegetable oil polyunsaturated fatty acid guinea pig skin delayed type hypersensitivity reaction properties", I have read some equally daunting nounal phrases.
> P B Medawar. *Advice to a Young Scientist*, Harper and Row, 1979

Nucleotides

Ebb and flow of the Irish Sea off Sellafield.

Nursery rhymes

Neglected educational medium. Contain relics not just of folklore and ancient incantations but of old reforming campaigns. Modern health educators have yet to tap in to this oral tradition.

> Jack and Jill
> Went down the pub
> And sank 10 pints of lager
> Jack fell down
> And broke his crown
> And Jill's completely gaga.
> *Medical Monitor.* 29, November 1991

Obituary prose

Coded language used in medical obituaries. Designed to provoke the reaction "Wasn't it well worth them dying to have that said of them" while conveying real meaning to *cognoscenti*.

John Rowan Wilson, custodian of the BMJ obituary column during the 1960s, compiled a glossary, since expanded by others:

A character	A tiresome old man
A perfectionist	An obsessional neurotic
Assertive	A bully
Plainspoken	Offensive
Did not suffer fools gladly	Damnably offensive
A man of strong opinions	A bigot
Charming	Dim but smiled a lot
Widely travelled	Left his juniors to do his work
Respected	Feared
One of the old school	Hopelessly out of date
Fond of the good things of life	A drunk
Had all the irresistible charm of the Celt	A talkative drunk

Obstetrical record

An award once held by Lucille Ball's husband.

> While Lucille was under contract to Harry Cohn at Colombia Pictures, she was loaned to Paramount for a De Mille picture *The Greatest Show on Earth*, but then discovered she was pregnant. De Mille sent a message to her husband: "Congratulations. You're the only man who's ever screwed his wife, Cecil B De Mille, Paramount Pictures, and Harry Cohn all at the same time".
> Looking sideways. *Medical Monitor*, 14 September 1990

Obvious

What learned journals put a lot of effort into explaining.

> Patients with chronic disease consult their general practitio-

ner frequently, and patients with more than one chronic disease consult even more frequently.

F G Schelleviset *et al.* Consultation rates and incidence of morbidity among patients with chronic disease in general practice.

British Journal of General Practice, June 1994

To manage changes effectively involves the ability to create a new synthesis of people, resources, ideas, opportunities, and demands.

Peter C Barnes. Managing change. *BMJ*, March 4 1995

Surprisingly 36% were stated to be alive up to one hour before death.

The Practitioner, May 1964

Off his trolley

Hospital slang for: "He has fallen out of his new improved NHS bed". *See* Bottomley ward.

Officiously to keep alive

Phrase used by casuists to protect themselves from difficult decisions about euthanasia. "Thou shalt not kill; but need'st not strive officiously to keep alive". Often quoted as the "correct" medical attitude by teachers who don't realise it comes from Arthur Hugh Clough's satirical reworking of the ten commandments to suit "market forces".

> Thou shalt have one God only; who
> Would be at the expense of two?
>
> Do not adultery commit;
> Advantage rarely comes of it.
>
> Thou shalt not steal; an empty feat,
> When it's so lucrative to cheat.
>
> Thou shalt not covet; but tradition
> Approves all forms of competition.
>
> Arthur Hugh Clough. *The Latest Decalogue*, 1862

Old scores

Carefully calculated debts that ambitious medical academics and politicians take great pleasure in paying off.

> As we grow older friends come and go but enemies accumulate.
>
> Cyril Chantler. *Personal communication*, 1996

> At times, when in depressive mood, I thought that far too much grudge harbouring went on in medicine. But then I was an editor—a potential ally for those with old scores to settle. I would remind myself that dermatologists probably think there's a lot of skin about, and chiropodists a lot of feet.
>
> World Medicine. A sort of obituary. *BMJ*, 3 October 1990

One more minute?

Traditional request to chairmen at scientific meetings from speakers who have already exceeded their allotted span by five minutes and intend to speak for another four. The only permissible response is: "I fear you are already trespassing on eternity".

Optimism

A healing quality. Beneficial both to patients and their doctors.

> Optimistic doctors help patients fight off the effects of disease and, at the same time, enhance their own reputations. When an optimist's patients die, relatives say: "The doctor was marvellous. He did all that was humanly possible but Nature beat him in the end". The pessimist's patients never die "despite his efforts". Even worse, they occasionally survive despite his efforts.
>
> There's a doctor close behind you. *An Insider's Guide to the Games Doctors Play*, Gollancz, 1986

> Optimism, I am convinced, is an essential component of that

ephemeral quality possessed by doctors whom patients feel better for seeing, no matter what treatment is prescribed. Such doctors are often assumed to be endowed with gifts denied to their colder hearted colleagues. But the "gift" is largely a technique.

A distinguished 19th century Dublin physician, Richard Leeper, used to tell his students: "Never give medicine to a dying man. Always give him brandy, for everyone knows that brandy never killed anyone. Give the patient medicine and someone will say: 'God forgive me if I wrong him, but Leeper's draught was the last thing the poor man took' ".

> On the run from Doctor Killjoy. *Times*, 3 July 1981

Out of hours commitment

Managerial euphemism for night calls.

> I can still 30 years later conjure up the insistent sound of the telephone ringing by my bed while I seek to convince myself it's only part of a dream and will disappear when I wake up. Yet once I was awake and the 'phone was still ringing, I knew before I lifted the receiver that I would have to visit the patient even if they asked only for advice. For if I didn't go I would just lie awake wondering if I'd done the right thing.
>
> *Heal thyself.* Radio Four, August 1995

> The general practitioners' newspaper *Pulse* recently had a competition for the worst night call. One of the winners was a GP who had been called at 1 am by a woman with asthma who had no inhaler. The GP visited, supplied a new inhaler, and made sure the attack had settled.
>
> "Thank you, doctor", she said as she saw him to the door. "My own inhaler is in my daughter's bedroom and I didn't want to wake her".
>
> Trisha Greenhalgh. *BMJ*, 9 September 1995

> The GP had barely settled back into bed after a night call when the 'phone rang again.
>
> "Sorry to bother you, doc", said a voice, "But I can't sleep. Is there anything you can do for me?"
>
> "Keep the phone to your ear", said the GP, "And I'll sing you a lullaby".
>
> *Monitor Weekly*, 22 June 1994

Over and Under

Dangerous words when used by bureaucrats who forget that each has a second meaning

> Child health surveillance consists of sets of activities initiated by professionals and includes the oversight of the physical, social and emotional health and development of all children.
> *Joint policy statement from the Berkshire FHSA, the Berkshire Health Authority and the East Berkshire Community Health Trust, 1993*

> Anne Macleod, who sent me a circular in which Clwyd FHSA encouraged GPs to set up Patient Participation Groups to help the "undeserving", thought they might mean "under-served" people but in the present political climate they could be in earnest.
> *Monitor Weekly*, 6 January 1994

Overflow (Trustspeak)

Displaced patients parked wherever there's room in the hospital.

> Mr X said that he and the surgeons were unhappy that the urological patients were overflowing into general surgical beds.
> Minutes of trust hospital management meeting.
> Anecdotal evidence. *Healthcare Management*, March 1994

Panglossism

Department of Health's attitude to its health promoting activities. Inspired by Dr Pangloss, philosopher and tutor in Voltaire's Candide—*dans ce meilleur des mondes possibles tout est au mieux* (all is for the best in the best of all possible worlds).

All those with a clear link between the reaction and the vaccine made a complete recovery; for children in whom recovery has been incomplete, there was no conclusive evidence to support an association with the vaccine.
CMO'S UPDATE 8, a communication to all doctors from the Chief Medical Officer, Department of Health, November 1995

Parameter

Verbal seasoning added to mundane statements to give them a flavour of erudition.

So "it is time the parameters were changed" to enable British industry to invest long-term (Leader, 25 July). Are these the same parameters that enabled Shane Warne "to operate within smaller parameters, with the line no longer such a give-away" (*Guardian*, 6 June 1993); or from which "adults cannot easily escape the parameters of their gender socialisation" (*Guardian*, 22 January 1994); or as the scientific discovery that will "change the parameters of science" (*Guardian*, 17 November 1992); or that occur "only within the parameters of current government thinking" (*Guardian*, 5 September 1992)?

I think the parameters (rules) of leader writing should be altered so that the parameters (subject matter) cannot exceed certain parameters (limits) or go beyond certain parameters (boundaries).
Dr Neville W Goodman. Letter to *Guardian*, 27 July 1995

Parental control, lack of

Antisocial behaviour in other people's children. As opposed to **hyperactivity**, antisocial behaviour in one's own children.

Parthenogenesis

A singular conception.

Partner

Near miss attempt to find neutral word for the other half of permanent or semipermanent relationship. Confusing when used by general practitioners

> Only last week when I was introduced to a GP and her partner, it took some delicate conversational probing to determine whether they shared a bed or an NHS list. Just to add to the confusion, it turned out they shared both.
> Looking sideways. *Medical Monitor*, 20 November 1992

> What term should we use? Lover suggests that the relationship is based only on sex and "live-in boyfriend or girlfriend" has too tabloid a ring. The only acceptable phrase I've encountered came from a Californian who introduced me to "the woman who shares my American Express card".
> Frank Giles, the former Fleet Street editor who married the daughter of an Earl, is an old hand at this naming game. Once when he received an invitation addressed to Mr and Mrs Giles he explained diffidently to his hostess over the 'phone that his wife wasn't exactly Mrs Giles. "Bring her along anyway", came the reply. "We're not stuffy about that sort of thing".
> *Ibid*

Pathography

Biography that exploits the experience of illness.

> The professional victim is one of the common guises of the pathographer. You know the sort of thing: someone, perhaps a celebrity, writes, or has ghost-written, a book about a real or self diagnosed illness, and then tours the talk shows and lecture circuit as an expert on victimhood. Luckily, expert victimhood is perfectly compatible with a life of wealthy hedonism.
> Bruce Charlton. *Theoretical Medicine*, 1995

> In practice, pathography is seen as an excuse to abandon self criticism, humility, stoicism, modesty, fortitude, good

143

manners, honesty and the whole caboodle—and as a licence to wallow in self pity, anger, tendentious reasoning, and self justification.

Ibid

They can be a good read. I remember enjoying George Pickering's *Creative Malady* in which he described how Florence Nightingale and Charles Darwin used their illnesses as social weapons. And he argued convincingly that psychoanalysis, *A la recherche du temps perdu*, and Christian Science owed their existence to attempts at self cure by Freud, Proust, and Mary Baker Eddy.

It will be a pity if the new wave of "tabloid" pathography drives out those honest accounts of illness "from the inside" that I've long believed can teach something to doctors and offer patients the sort of support they get from self help groups.

Medical Monitor, 7 February 1995

Patient choice

Empowering critically ill patients to choose between being shunted round the country in search of a bed or going home to die.

An urgent review of hospital intensive care facilities was ordered by the Government yesterday after a nationwide survey disclosed serious shortages of beds. In some areas, up to half of all such patients referred to hospital are refused admission.

A separate survey by doctors at St George's Hospital, in Tooting, south west London, reported that intensive care units were frequently full, forcing the transfer by ambulance of critically ill patients to any hospital that could take them...

Some of the rejected patients had a 50% higher chance of dying than some of those who got a bed, the study found.

News report. *Daily Telegraph*, 8 February 1995

Patients

Quirky individuals whose idiosyncrasies disrupt well ordered professional lives.

144

[Literary] agents are like doctors: they prefer dealing with one another. Clients, like patients, are secondary—there to be soothed and comforted and lied to while the real business is done in straight talking between professional men. This is after all what a professional man is: someone who can talk to other professional men without feeling or feeling only a precise measure of concern that will pass for feeling. This is why voters distrust politicians, a prisoner his lawyer, and, at this particular moment, why I am unhappy with my agent.

Alan Bennett. *Writing Home*, Faber, 1994

Patients' best interests

Phrase doctors use to justify pursuing their own.

Patient's charter

A device for diverting money from the care of patients to the sustenance of government supporters in the public relations, advertising, and glossy paper industries.

It's easy to understand Dr Robert Addlestone's disbelief when he dropped in at his local Lawnswood crematorium in Leeds and picked up a booklet entitled *The Dead Citizen's Charter*.

Not only was it written in deadly earnest—if you'll pardon the expression—but was described by its authors as "a consultative document". And like most citizen's charters its opening sentence was designed to reveal one of those great truths that we would never have discovered for ourselves: "An individual's funeral will take place just once".

Medical Monitor, 27 November 1996

Patients' needs

Weasel phrase that allows authorities to decide what people should be allowed to have.

The word "need" has been used to mean two different things:

- A way in which someone's life falls short of what they

might reasonably hope for, and
- A requirement for a service, which has been accepted by the body responsible for providing it.

Only the second of these should be called a "need". The first should be called a "problem".

Newsletter for people working in community social and health services in Northumberland.

Quoted in *Medical Monitor*, 8 September 1993

I have rights
You have needs
He has problems

Medical Monitor, 8 September 1993

Pedagoguery

Teaching role that some doctors regard as synonymous with demagoguery.

David Jobling, a GP in Knaresborough, received this letter from a consultant.

"This gentleman did not attend for his appointment today. A DNA is certainly a risk factor for a large psychological element to a chronic pain.

I would, however, advise you to guard against the mistake of relying on classical Cartesian mind/body dualism when dealing with chronic pain problems. It is now clear that the mind resides in the brain and the brain functions by being an adaptive network of nerves. This adaptation occurs not just in the brain, but throughout the nervous system extending to the tips of C fibre endings.

This can not only affect nerve function, but also things like erythema and swelling around the site of injury, all under neural control. It is therefore very unclear where the mind ends and the body begins, or vice-versa".

Dr Jobling claimed to be impressed by such fulsome advice about a patient who hadn't even attended the clinic

Medical Monitor, 20 March 1996

Performance

GMCspeak for competence. Accusing doctors of "poor performance" is less likely to upset their political representatives than calling them incompetent.

Personal development

Elusive yet profitable commodity that NHS management consultants try to sell to the insecure. The first step is to clog the mind with pretentious phrases.

> GPs in the fiefdom of the South Western Regional Health Authority have been invited to spend £300 to discover how to create "a culture of empowerment" by attending a programme that used "development centre techniques to enhance the learning process". The invitation describes the techniques in a characteristic paragraph:
>
> "The programme incorporates objective, competency based rating procedures, and the use of practical, work related exercises. Strengths and development needs are identified and feedback is based on observed behaviour. The focus is on the individual, and participants evaluate their own performance and define the key objectives associated with their role. The competency framework and rating procedure is easy to understand and the combination of self and peer assessment ensures that feedback is based on two way discussion, and learning points fully incorporated in Action Plans".
>
> So there.
>
> Anecdotal evidence. *Healthcare Management*, May 1994

Perversions

One's own shameful fantasies acted out by others.

Phonetic diagnosis

Ideally suited to a market-led NHS—but dangerous.

> Patients being admitted to one of London's newest trust hospitals have to answer a comprehensive questionnaire that covers not just traditional ground—occupation, next of kin, and so on— but a detailed family history and a series "lifestyle" questions devised by a "health marketing" whiz kid.
>
> A woman who recently survived this interrogation was puzzled when it came to an end. "You've asked all these

questions about my relatives and friends", she said, "Yet asked nothing at all about my husband and children?"

"That's because of your occupation", said the admissions clerk, snapping the folder shut. Only when the woman thought back did she remember that when asked her occupation she'd answered: "None".
Looking sideways. *Medical Monitor*, 1 May 1992

Placebo

Most effective medication known to science. Subjected to more clinical trials than any other. Nearly always does better than anticipated. Range of susceptible conditions appears to be limitless. Valued by clinicians but under-rated by pharmacologists who see its range and flexibility as a threat to their discoveries.

Any doctor fool enough to think that patients are passively obedient should recall that memorable clinical trial in which the subjects broke the code by discovering that when they threw their tablets down the lavatory, the drug floated but the placebo sank.
Compliance. *BMA News Review*, October 1990

Politically inept

Any action or statement that a doctor fears will upset those who control patronage and preferment within the profession. *See* Gravitas and Decent chap.

Postmortem examination

An occasion when a pathologist can tell a surgeon where he or she went wrong. (And when a surgeon can point out that the pathologist works through a somewhat larger incision.)

Precocious puberty

Puberty in other people's daughters.

Prescription

Originally a device for ensuring that a patient would pay another visit to the doctor. Now recognised as a component of the mystical process of healing.

> The custom of prescribing some medicine for every illness, even when it is not necessary, is equivalent to magic, especially when the prescription is written, as it once was, in Latin or in indecipherable handwriting. Most prescriptions would be just as effective if they were not taken to the druggist, but were simply hung on a string around the patient's neck.
>
> Carlo Levi. *Christ Stopped at Eboli*, Cassell, 1948

Prison

Traditional 19th century treatment for mental illness revived in the last decade of 20th century.

> A schizophrenia sufferer who killed two people after his release from hospital has been sent to prison because a judge said sending him to secure hospital could not guarantee public safety. Judge Peter Beaumont rejected psychiatrists' recommendations that Wayne Hutchinson be sent to Broadmoor for treatment and instead insisted he be sent to prison. Mr Hutchinson was released from the Southwestern Hospital in Brixton by mistake in 1994. Judge Beaumont argued that if he were sent to a mental hospital again, he might be released after a short time if his condition was judged to have improved.
>
> News report. *Independent*, 2 February 1996

> A teenager with the mental age of 10 has been held on remand in Exeter prison for two months because his local health authority was unable to find him a place in a secure psychiatric unit.
>
> The lawyer representing Christopher Saunders, 18, from Plymouth, claims that since his incarceration his already unstable mental condition has deteriorated. His mother, Rosie Saunders, claims her son, who was recently diagnosed as a paranoid psychotic, has lost weight and is unable to cope with being left alone for hours on end. He was

remanded on February 17 by Plymouth magistrates after being charged with five counts of assault and one of criminal damage.

News report. *Guardian*, 9 April 1997

Probity gap

Political malaise of the 1990s. The chasm that lies between what we're told is happening and our everyday experience.

Consultant dermatologist Angus Macdonald suspects an entry has gone missing from our dictionaries. "There must be a specific word or phrase", he writes, "To express the act of persuading people that things are getting better simply by altering the goal posts or shuffling the tables and chairs. This would describe the process whereby we are all told continually that as a result of charters, etc, the NHS is improving while all of us working within it know this is not the case".

Anecdotal evidence. *Medical Interface*, April 1997

In a recent issue, the *Sunday Telegraph*'s editor Dominic Lawson described a dinner party at which his wife sat next to a Tory member of the Commons Select Health Committee.

Her neighbour, according to Lawson, is "one of the ablest MPs of the younger generation" and when Mrs L embarked on fiery condemnation of mixed-sex hospital wards, he assured her that they no longer existed. When she persisted, the MP's manner, according to Mr L, slipped from good humoured condescension to strained patience: "No, no, no. You are quite wrong. It is all in the Patient's Charter. There are no more mixed wards in the NHS. We've phased them out". Whereupon Mrs Lawson revealed that she had recently been a patient in a mixed ward at St Mary's, Paddington, and described in graphic detail the indignities to which she'd been subjected.

Describing the incident Lawson suggested it could have been the vividness of those details that "finally convinced the Tory MP that the NHS mixed ward really did still exist despite all the statements to the contrary made by Government ministers to his committee".

Which makes one wonder whether this "ablest" of health committee members ever speaks to real doctors and nurses—let me rephrase that—ever listens to real doctors and nurses. Or does he, as has become the custom, consult only with the faithful?

Anecdotal evidence. *Medical Interface*, January 1996

Professional ambiguity

The art of making unambiguous comment in testimonials and book reviews

> I've never quite had the guts to use the testimonial said to have been written by Noel Glover, the Guy's surgeon who taught me in the 1960s: "You will be lucky to get this man to work for you".
>
> Richard Newell, Penarth surgeon. *Personal communication*

> Recently, when we were discussing the difficulty of writing testimonials, an orthopaedic surgeon showed me one he'd received about a man who'd applied to be his registrar. It ended: "He conceals his true character beneath a civilised veneer that is soluble in alcohol".
>
> Looking sideways. *Medical Monitor*, 26 April 1991

> Lord Walton, bless him, tells you everything you never wanted to know about the rise and rise of a lad from Spennymoor to the heights of the medical trade (professor of neurology, president of the BMA (twice), chairman of the GMC, warden of Green College, etc, etc,), not failing to mention that his mother's mother was well cared for by a companion called Mabel, that he spent much time in the church choir hoping for a glimpse of his future wife's knees as she swung round on the organ stool, that his elder daughter was a wakeful baby, that Dulwich has a splendid picture gallery and Lichtenstein lovely mountain scenery, that Holland is flat, and that in 1963 he and Betty (of the knees) while house hunting in Newcastle found that several "were attractive but had significant disadvantages, even including some in Elmfield and in Graham Park Road".
>
> Ruth Holland. Review of The Spice of Life: From Northumbria to World Neurology by John Walton.
> *BMJ*, 23 October 1993

> A doctor novelist of my acquaintance who is plagued with unsolicited manuscripts, always replies politely: "Thank you for sending me your book. I shall lose no time in

reading it".

Anecdotal evidence. *Medical Interface*, April 1966

Prognosis

A guess that some doctors make with extraordinary precision. "His doctors gave him six months to live". Successful prognosticators give details only to suggestible patients and deliver them in firm dogmatic tones.

> You will feel "under the weather" for two weeks. Then will come four weeks in which you will feel fit but be short of energy and of enthusiasm to do things. Don't despair. After six weeks you will wake up magically one morning and discover you are back to being your old self.
> *Leaflet handed to patients by a London urologist, 1986*

> The world is full of gleeful old fogies eager to describe how they cheated their pessimistic doctors. They wave their walking sticks and tell us proudly how, maybe 40 years before, some gloomy killjoy gave them only six months to live.
> There's a doctor close behind you. *An Insider's Guide to the Games Doctors Play*, Gollancz, 1986

> The most effective use of medical notes I ever came across was that deployed by a gynaecologist who built a profitable reputation for forecasting the sex of unborn babies. He told each pregnant woman that she was going to have a boy, but wrote girl in the notes.
> If his patient delivered a girl, he showed her the notes written in her presence and explained that she must have misheard.
> Health warning: doctors' notes are bad for the ego.
> *Times*, 4 September 1981

Promiscuity

Undefined term used by those who would protect us from ourselves.

> In the 18th century, frequent coition was blamed for

innumerable ills. Nicolas Venette, an eminent French surgeon, in his widely read *Tableau de l'amour conjugal* (translated into English in 1750), listed the brain melting like ice before the fire, eyes growing dim, consumption, diabetes, loss of hair and memory, shortening of one's life by two thirds, as some of the consequences of venereal excess.

Sex in moderation, on the other hand, was wholesome, clearing one's mind and eyesight, and protecting against epilepsy, gout and green sickness; in fact there was "no surer or safer means to preserve health and avoid sudden death than now and then to take a frick with a woman". It was all a matter of deciding the correct interpretation of "now and then".

Petr Skrabanek. *The Death of Humane Medicine and the Rise of Coercive Healthism*, The Social Affairs Unit, 1994
[Skrabanek suggests a rule of thumb definition of promiscuity
—having more partners than the user of the word.]

Providing a better service

Phrase used by health ministers when closing Accident and Emergency departments, reducing hospital beds, cutting the number of doctors and nurses, closing hospitals, or indeed doing anything likely to produce a worse service.

Pseudoparentalism

Attitude sometimes adopted by the young towards those they assume are in their "second childhood".

Dear Doctor, Could you please call and see my mother who has taken to going out on walks on her own though she's now 65.
Note received by Surrey GP, 1993

He told me of a family that lived near to him in Philadelphia—a household consisting of husband and wife, three adolescent daughters, and the husband's widowed 80 year old mother. The family worried that the old lady rarely got out of the house so they arranged a "date" for her with a widower who lived nearby and was also in his 80s.

153

She was very late getting home and the whole family had
to sit up to wait for her. When she came in, her son asked
anxiously: "Did you have a good time?"
"Are you kidding?" snapped his mother. "I had to slap his
face three times".
"Gosh", said one of the granddaughters. "Did he try to get
fresh?"
"No", said the old lady. "I thought he was dead".

Monitor Weekly, 31 May 1995

Psychspeak

Obfuscatory language developed by those who like to invest their
speculation about the working of the human mind with an aura of
authority.

He has developed insight regarding factors which pre-
cipated his islets of verbal dyscontrol and he has begun to
utilise his emotional gearbox particularly his brakes appro-
priately.

Clinical psychologist's letter to Paul Mason,
a Weymouth GP, 1994

The verbal group therapies include client-centred counselling and insight-oriented psychotherapy. Definitive features
of these modalities are discussion of the patients' problems
and mobilisation of member-to-member and member-to-
therapist interaction to improve psycho-behavioral
functioning.
Christine V. Abramowitz. The effectiveness of group
psychotherapy with children. *Archives of General*
Psychiatry, March 1976

Her spontaneous replies from unconscious sources within
her indicate that the therapeutic goal of reorienting a portion
of herself that has been so frantically and anxiously
dependent upon outside sources of support has been
responding to, accepting and depending upon internal
sources of wisdom and strength and that this has lessened
the panic coming from this source, and has also given the

self a means of internal influence upon the formerly uncontrollable anxiety.

Psychiatric report quoted by Edmund J Simpson. Verba sesquipedalia.

Journal of the American Medical Association,
20 January 1969
[Simpson wonders if this is a sentence.
"Every time I look for a verb I get a headache".]

Public opinion

Elusive entity more often invoked than measured. Mother phrase of others like "silent majority" or "all right-thinking people".

In a series of interviews based on a questionnaire, a last question was added as an impish afterthought.
You have just given me your opinion on a number of topics to do with medicine and medical research. Do you think your opinions:
(a) Generally reflect public opinion on these matters
(b) Differ from public opinion on these matters
(c) You don't know.
  You may be as delighted as I was to discover that only 22% of the 200 respondents thought their ideas reflected public opinion, 70% thought their opinion differed from public opinion, and 8% didn't know.
The demands of public opinion. *Constraints on the advance of medicine, proceedings of RSM,* December 1974

Publish or perish

Cardinal principle of academia. A choice between fame and oblivion. Most academics find it difficult to handle either gracefully.

Pudder

Term coined by Ivor Brown for a style of writing that expresses meaning in as complicated a way as possible. Lingua franca of a **scientific paper**.

Experiments are described which demonstrate that in

normal individuals the lowest concentration in which sucrose can be detected by means of gustation differs from the lowest concentration in which sucrose (in the amount employed) has to be ingested in order to produce a demonstrable decrease in olfactory acuity and a noteworthy conversion of sensations interpreted as a desire for food into sensations interpreted as satiety associated with ingestion of foods.

C Mawdsley. Medical pudder. Res Medica, 1968

Let us describe a bow legged man.

In pudder we could say: "The patient has a marked varus deformity of the lower extremities of rachitic aetiology".

Plain speaking, plus a little rhythm and rhyme might render this as: "Over the hill and down the road, comes a man whose legs are bowed". Add drama and we have: "Oh what manner of man is this with testes in parenthesis?"

Ibid

Pull through

Enigmatic act that patients are alleged to perform when they recover.

Begs three questions:
- Pull though what?
- On what do the pullers achieve the necessary purchase?
- Is the doctor's job to push or to assist the pull?

Punitive medicine

Treatment based on the premise that people often need "a good shake up" to "bring them back to their senses".

This 16 year old girl is suffering from hysterical epilepsy as a result of seeing a fit at a football match. I think I have cured her by a firm talk. I told her mother that, if they recur, she should smack her face and pour cold water over her.

Letter from a consultant at the Bristol Royal Infirmary, 1954. Quoted in *Healthcare Management*, March 1995

Back in the 1970s, John Rowan Wilson and I took an interest in punitive medicine, inspired as I recall by S J Perelman's suggestion that the most effective way to control thumb sucking was to nail the infant's hands to the side of the cot.

One of John's ripest discoveries was in a book generally regarded as a medical classic, indeed one highly recommended to my generation of medical students by teachers desperate to give us a veneer of erudition: *Hilton's Rest and Pain.*

A condition that caused Hilton grave concern was masturbation—or, as he preferred it, onanism—which he regarded as a source of much serious illness. He admitted it was "a habit very difficult to contend with in practice", assumed it afflicted only males, and recommended painting the victim's penis with a strong tincture of iodine to ensure that it blistered and became so sore that the patient could not bear to touch it.

Anecdotal evidence. *Healthcare Management*, March 1995

Pursuing an improper sexual relationship

GMCspeak for a sexual adventure between a doctor and a patient, or between a doctor and a nurse, or between doctors and any other persons they may meet in the course of their work. A charge rarely made when the pursuit is in full cry. Usually made by the non-doctor after the affair has come to an unhappy end.

The fact that many doctors marry nurses, and that some marry their patients, suggests a lot of improper pursuing goes on early in medical careers.

> I'm puzzled by one phrase you used. Pursuing an improper sexual relationship, I think it was. Does the adjective "improper" imply there are proper techniques to which we should have restricted ourselves—certain positions maybe that we should have adopted? If so, I have to plead ignorance to what constitutes propriety in these matters.
>
> *Serious Professional Misconduct*, (In press)

Qualification

Mysterious process alleged to transmute the traditionally raffish medical student into a wise, trustworthy, and kindly physician.

> His low opinion of medical students sprang largely from the days when he had been reading Theology at Cambridge and, on his attempt to break up a noisy party of medicals late one night, he had been forcibly administered an enema of Guinness stout.
>
> Richard Gordon. *Doctor in the House*, Michael Joseph, 1948

> Only last night a figure from my past appeared as an "expert" on my television screen. When we were students no one would trust him with the price of a drink, not to mention the address of a girlfriend. Yet there he was last night telling me why every 15 year old girl should or shouldn't be on the Pill; I forget which it was but he said it with great authority.
>
> One man's burden. *BMJ*, 3 August 1985

Quality

(Noun) A medical attribute that can be discerned only by senior colleagues. Hence the conjugation: "I have quality, you are competent, he needs auditing".

(Adj.) Trustspeakers' favourite modifier: quality care, total quality management, etc.

Quality of life

A judgment doctors consider themselves capable of making about other people's lives. When used in rationing decisions, becomes a judgment of other people's worth.

> Those whose lives could have been judged as of little worth include indubitable loonies like Vincent van Gogh, hopeless drunks like Scott Fitzgerald and Dylan Thomas, and the

"seriously handicapped" like Christy Brown and Stephen Hawking.

Stop the Week. BBC Radio 4, January 1991

When my elderly mother was ill last year, the specialist informed me that she would soon die and there was nothing he would do. However, if her "quality of life" had been better, he said—if, say, her husband had been alive—then the situation would be different and he might come to another decision. I am not arguing with his decision, but as he broke the news I wondered for a moment what right an expert in removing intestines had to be an expert on someone's "quality of life".

Peter Hillmore. *Observer,* 24 March 1997

Rationing

Protecting your own resources while stealing those belonging to others.

You quote the OPCS study as reporting that Manchester is the least healthy place for men in England. Last week, the Department of Health released the allocation to health authorities in England. All received growth funding bar two: Camden and Islington, and Manchester. Manchester was deemed to be overfunded for the health needs of its residents. The OPCS is run by the Department of Health

Chris Jeffries, Cheadle Hulme, Cheshire.

Letter to *Guardian,* 11 December 1995

After our government turned our NHS into a market place, it became fashionable for politicians and NHS administrators to visit the State of Oregon, which had initiated not only public debate of rationing but public decision on its implementation. Indeed Oregon became one of those words you needed to drop into a lecture or a paper just to show you were one of the brave new thinkers.

Yet not one of the many commendatory articles that visitors wrote on their return mentioned that in the State of Oregon 120 000 children still have no access to any sort of health care.

Medical Monitor, 12 June 1996

Reaccreditation

Disgraceful bureaucratic assault on the status of those who are already fully trained.

> My original certification was based on holding bachelor of medicine and bachelor of surgery qualifications and this in turn was based on knowing the chemical formula for soap and that exhibit 24a was a uterine fibroid. Later I could have spent six months in an approved post learning and practising little more than phlebotomy.
> The testing of actual performance in general practice is a quantum step forward from my certification experience and, as a measure of the delivery of health care, is something we as general practitioners should welcome now; it is certainly what the justification of our professional future will soon hinge on.
> A J Dow. Letter: *British Journal of General Practice*,
> December 1995

Reader deterrence

Invaluable bureaucratic "written communications" skill. Ensures readers retire baffled before completing the first paragraph.

> A letter from Camidoc, otherwise known as the Camden & Islington Doctors On-call Co-operative, to Fred Kavalier, GP of that parish:
> "It is now an accepted requirement that all out of hours providers have in place a routine and developed structure for the monitoring of procedural action times for all received calls on the system. In effect, this means that Camidoc staff must detail [for the Health Authority] the specific time of each separate action on behalf of any patient call as it passes through our developed system ..." etc, etc.
> *Medical Monitor*, 5 March 1997

> Barely had I announced my institution of a Diploma in Reader Deterrence when a queue of applicants formed at my door. At their head was Denzil Jones of the Welsh Office who recently sent a "clarifying" note to the long suffering GPs of the Principality. Here's his diploma-winning paragraph:

"I will start by confirming the position for patient costs. Here we have drawn a distinction between reimbursing transport costs to enable a patient to avail him or herself of NHS Services, and reimbursement for transport costs where a patient is availing him or herself of such services. Where there is determined to be a medical need for transport it can be said that the patient is availing him or herself of NHS Services when transport is provided".

I assure you it gets little better as it goes on.

Medical Monitor, 2 April 1997

Reflex riposte centre

Clutch of cells in mid-brain that can cope with massive sensory input and produce an instant yet entertaining motor response without apparent intervention from higher centres. In a true riposte reflex the gap between stimulation and response allows no time for cerebration and the riposte is as much a surprise to its utterer as to its provoker.

When the surgeon/novelist John Rowan Wilson was asked by an editor the meaning of Mons Veneris, he replied instantly "Fanny Hill".

Medical Monitor, 29 January 1993

When a member of *World Medicine*'s advertising department, who'd been reading more of the journal than was good for him, sidled up to the editor and asked what one of the contributors meant by "the lateral coital position", the editor heard his voice reply, even before the question was completed: "Having a bit on the side".

Ibid

Frank Muir and Denis Norden have often made me contemplate the physiology of repartee. Do their minds flash tangentially in search of ideas? Or do they have accelerated retrieval of lines they wrote years ago. Whatever the answer, the result is impressive.

During a recent recording of My Word, after we'd been dealing with some item of history, I asked Frank, without warning, what historical incident he would like to have witnessed. He paused for but a moment before replying: "I'd like to have been present at the destruction of the cities of the plain. I've always wanted to know, doctor, what went on in Gomorrah?"

Looking sideways. *Medical Monitor*, 20 July 1990

Refurbishment (Trustspeak)

Deploying resources on tarting up premises rather than on what takes place within them.

A consultant recently took early retirement rather than move his department into the new premises that, after years of broken promises, his masters had eventually provided. "You may think I'm mad", he said, "But after spending my entire professional life practising 20th century medicine in 19th century surroundings I didn't want to spend the last two years in unfamiliar territory".

I assured him that if he were mad, it was a common form of loopiness. I told him of the evening Sir Seymour Hicks, the actor manager, entered the lavatory at the Garrick Club and discovered that, while he'd been on tour, it had been lavishly redecorated. As he stood at the urinal, the man in the next stall gazed around the new surroundings and said: "Impressive, isn't it?" "Indeed", said Seymour Hicks, "But it does make the old prick look a bit shabby".

Anecdotal evidence. *Healthcare Management*, April 1995

Relationships

Human alliances that doctors seek to explain but rarely understand.

In the pre-pill days, I remember one of my partners attending a hazardous home delivery. When the deed was safely done, he said to the mother "This is the seventh child you've had by this man. Why don't you marry him?"

"Oh I could never do that doctor".

"Don't you think you owe it to the children, if not to yourself?"

"Maybe. But I could never marry him, doctor".

"Why not?"

"Because I've never really liked him".

Medical Monitor, 2 October 1996

Repetitive strain injury

A disease of prose. Syntactical damage caused by overemphasis. Severe attacks can cause serious loss of meaning.

> In addition, there has been bouts and bouts of intermittent variable periods of fluctuations of ups and downs.
>> Letter dictated by Hertfordshire doctor. Quoted by David Delvin, *BMA News Review*, 5 February 1997

> It is considered that this could be significant even though not at present but now.
> Medical report quoted by Edmund J Simpson, *Journal of the American Medical Association*, 20 January 1969

Research

What I do for the benefit of humanity, you do for the money, and he does for the publicity.

Resentful Prisoner Syndrome

Fate of many doctors who are good at their job and extract most of the personal satisfaction from it by their late 30s. They then grow bored and turn their hands to dangerous activities like politics or administration. *See* Career structures.

> When I first wrote about the syndrome, the letters came not singly but in sackfuls. Most were from clinicians whose attitude to their work had run a similar course: excitement, enthusiasm, and involvement in the early days; boredom entering their lives insidiously and, at first, un-noticed as they entered their late 30s. Finally came recognition and acknowledgement of the boredom and a depressing feeling of imprisonment within a career that offered little flexibility and from which the only escape was that distant pension.
>> One man's burden. *BMJ*, 22 January 1983

> One day David Connell, who had been a general practitioner in Berkshire for 16 years, conjured up a vision of himself as an old man. His grandson sat on his knee and

asked: "Grandpa, what did you do with your life?" and he heard himself reply: "I went to medical school, qualified as a doctor, worked in a hospital for a year or two, then settled down as a family doctor in this pleasant town for 40 years". The vision horrified him.

One man's burden. *BMJ*, 3 December 1983

A career in medicine should continually broaden an intelligent person's vision rather than restrict it. Anton Chekov wrote: "My medical colleagues sigh with envy when they meet me and talk about literature and say how sick and tired they are of medicine. The strange thing is that medicine has had a great influence on my literary work. It has widened the field of my observation and enriched my knowledge". Postgraduate education needs to free the resentful prisoners by promoting enrichment at the expense of disenchantment.

The resentful prisoner game. *An Insider's Guide to the Games Doctors Play*, Gollancz, 1986

Resignation

1. A state of mind which helps younger doctors come to terms with the NHS reforms.
2. An act which helps older doctors do the same.

Responsible (Trustspeak)

Not accountable.

The father of Georgina Robinson, the occupational therapist who was stabbed to death by a mentally ill patient on unsupervised leave from Torbay's Edith Morgan Centre, has called for the resignation of three managers. But South Devon healthcare trust chief executive Tony Parr, chair Tony Boyce, and director of nursing Hilary Cunliffe, are all staying put. As Mr Boyce put it: "There will be no disciplinary action or resignation at board level. Everybody accepts responsibility for what happened".

Doing the rounds. *Private Eye*, 27 January 1995

Reunions

Occasions organised by medical schools to give contemporaries a chance to assess their relative decrepitude.

> When he was dean of the medical school, the sons of many of his contemporaries had come for interviews. He recognised them immediately because they looked like their fathers and had the same attitudes and mannerisms as their fathers. Only when he met the parents did he realise that the fathers no longer looked like the fathers.
>
> *Medical Monitor*, 29 January 1993

Rhetorical pronouns

Two little words used by politicians when discussing the NHS.

We
Used when things are going well.

> We are now doing many more hip operations than we did 10 years ago.
>
> Virginia Bottomley.
> *Jonathan Dimbleby*, ITV, 23 April 1995

They
Used when things are going badly.

> They have not yet managed to get their priorities right in that hospital.
>
> *Ibid*

Risk

Like most ideas about gambling, a wholly irrational concept.

> Sir Herman Bondi, the mathematician, described a Swedish plan to study the Aurora Borealis by firing instrument-carrying rockets into it. When the rockets had done their job, the burnt out remnants fell over a sparsely populated area of Lapland. To prevent injury, the government flew out

the only residents, a handful of reindeer herders, by helicopter. The probability of one of them being hit by a piece of rocket was less than 1% of that of a helicopter accident but the action can be justified—politically if not mathematically.

If someone had been hit, the Interior Minister would have been accused of doing nothing to protect the Lapps. Yet, if a helicopter had crashed, people would have accepted a statement that said: "We offer our deepest sympathy to the relatives of the victims. We used a well-tried helicopter, flown by an experienced crew. We are appalled by what happened but there is no other precaution we could have taken". Whatever the mathematicians might have said, it would have been an Act of God.

Lecture. *Edinburgh Science Festival*, April 1993

On 15 July 1992 the broadsheets carried front page reports that the antihistamine Triludan had caused cardiac arrhythmias in six patients who had either exceeded the recommended dose or taken it with erythromycin.

On the same morning, the *Independent*'s diary, reported that "at least two US soldiers die each year as a result of kicking faulty vending machines". And another 25 GIs are injured after "kicking, striking, shaking or otherwise assaulting malfunctioning vending machines which in consequence fall over".

A nice diary piece. Good for a laugh. Yet the laughably minute risk of being killed by a vending machine is at least 200 times greater than the "drug scare" risk presented in stark solemnity on the front page.

Looking sideways. *Medical Monitor*, 31 July 1992

Road glee

Psychopathy induced by congested traffic. Commoner than road rage but less well publicised.

The town of Reading, I'm reliably informed, is known for its competitive motorists and one of the patients seen in the local A&E over Christmas was a pedestrian knocked down by a hit-and-run driver. Luckily he wasn't badly injured and as the houseman wrote up the notes he heard a policeman ask his patient if he'd noticed the licence number of the car that struck him.

"No", came the reply, "But I'd remember his laugh anywhere".

Roost (BMAspeak)

Where the chickens will come home to.

Royal Free Tubing Fallacy, the

Medical jargon for any nonsensical suggestion that seems wholly logical to a bureaucratic mind. Named after a management decision minuted at the Royal Free Hospital, London, in November 1976.

> The minute reads: "a request was made for more stethoscopes in A/E. It was not felt that this was possible but it was suggested that longer tubing be put onto the existing ones in the department".
> *Medical Monitor*, 17 March 1993

> In our Department meeting we have agreed that results will be sent out promptly and other results you are waiting for can be sent out separately at a later date.
> *Hospital communication sent to Bradford GP David Fieldhouse*, 1993

Sanctimony

Air of piety sometimes affected by doctors who specialise in treatment of the rich.

> Dr Bodkin Adams, an Eastbourne GP, was charged with poisoning elderly women after he'd induced them to include him in their wills.
> Sometimes when he entered a house Adams would drop

dramatically to his knees and pray for the patient he was about to see. The younger sister of one of his patients described at his trial what happened one day after she had admitted him at the front door and started to lead him upstairs to the sick-room. She was less than halfway when she heard the doctor call out behind her and there was a loud crash. When she turned she saw him lying on the floor of the hall. According to her evidence, he explained that when he knelt on a mat to pray for the sick woman's recovery it slipped from under him on the polished floor.

Counsel asked: "Could you hear what Dr Adams called out as he fell?"

The witness said, "Yes. He shouted, 'oh fuck'.

Anecdotal evidence. *Healthcare Management*, June 1993

Saniflush

All-conquering concept of psychotherapy. Popular in California.

Bruce Sloame, a British expatriate psychiatrist working in Los Angeles, once convinced me that the local enthusiasm for cosmetic surgery, and indeed for psychoanalysis, derived from what he called the Saniflush concept of psychotherapy—a belief that we all have it within ourselves to achieve greatness if only some therapist or guru could flush out the hang ups that get in the way.

Audiomonitor, June 1995

Science

Subversion.

Ask an impertinent question! That is the essence of science.

Jacob Bronowski.
Nature and Knowledge, Random House,1969

Science is a mosaic of partial and conflicting visions. But there is one common element in these visions. The common element is rebellion against the restrictions imposed by the locally prevailing culture.

F Dyson. The scientist as rebel.
The New York Review of Books, May 1995

Semanticist Paul Lippert recently pointed out that in many societies there has persisted an irritating group of people who are in the habit of asking more questions than they answer. They are called by various names: artists, philosophers, troublemakers. In the Middle Ages, some of these irksome people caused quite a stir, but enough time has now passed so that we call them scientists.

William A Silverman. *Pediatric Pathology*, vol 1, 1983

Sciencespiel

Form of **Decorated Municipal Gothic** (DMG) that writers have to use to get scientific papers published.

Here, to give you a taste, are just a few scientifically correct DMG words. You'll have no problem constructing a glossary of your own. Just read a paper or two in any journal.

DMG	Translation
Facilitate	Ease
Numerous	Many
General public	People
Public at large	People
Initial	First
Remainder	Rest
Implement	Do
Utilise	Use
Locate	Find
Transmit	Send
Majority of	Most

Let just one of these words into a paper, or a lecture, and the infection will spread with the abandon of organisms that have alighted on a nutrient medium.

The toxic effect of language on medicine. *Journal of the Royal College of Physicians of London*, November/December 1995

We need to restore a literary tradition in medicine, a tradition in which language is used not just to pass on information but to stimulate the imagination, to provoke thought, and to encourage the creativity that too easily gets swamped in a morass of data.

Ibid

Scientific method

Accepted by doctors to be a good thing though they're not quite sure what it is.

> There is an assumption that if you go through the motions of science then science will result. Many of the efforts remind one of the experiments that children perform with chemistry sets: "Follow instructions and you can be a real chemist just like the picture on the box".
> Erving Goffman. *Relations in Public*, Basic Books, 1971

> Soon after acquiring a PhD in one of the more exact sciences, he was appointed "scientist to the surgical unit" at a London teaching hospital. When asked what the job entailed, he used to say: "The professor removes a piece of tissue, gives it to me, and expects me to go off and do something scientific with it".
> One man's burden. *BMJ*, 17 August 1985

Scientific paper

Piece of ill written prose that serves many worthy purposes save that for which it claims to exist—the passing on of information. *See* Literature, Understanding.

> [Scientific papers] represent the productivity and therefore the "value" of the research team; they establish hierarchies by the ordering of their author lines and by whom they chose to cite; and, most importantly of all, they stake their author's claim to the new knowledge they contain. They serve the needs of their authors above the needs of their readers.
> Michael Shortland, Jane Gregory.
> *Communicating Science: A Handbook*, Longman, 1991

Scruffie's Triangle

Significant anatomical site for doctors in search of increased productivity. Named after Dr Ignatius Scruffie, productivity pioneer of the 1950s and '60s who ministered to vast numbers of the sick from the front parlour of a terrace house highly adjacent to the Slagthorpe marshalling yards.

"Let me teach you an important piece of clinical anatomy", said Ignatius. He undid a button midway down his shirt front and pulled the material an inch to one side. "See that gap, my lad? That's Scruffie's Triangle. Whenever you see a patient who's concerned about a cough, or palpitations or a weak heart, expose the Triangle, plonk your stethoscope in the middle of it, listen learnedly for 30 seconds, then tell them there's nothing to worry about. It works wonders".
Looking sideways. *World Medicine*, 16 May 1967

Ignatius always maintained that auscultating the Triangle was a safe procedure. Patients who were really ill, he said, would soon return and could then be dispatched to the Slagthorpe Memorial with one of his visiting cards that not only had his name and address on the front but a printed message to the Casualty Officer on the back: *Please Examine*.
Audiomonitor, January 1997

Ignatius Scruffie's contemporary "Wee Willie" McAnny of Slagcliffe-le-Willows described a similar area that was exposed when women patients placed the fingers of both hands in the neckline of their dress or jumper and pulled down for an inch and a half. This is known as McAnny's Rhomboid Space.
Daily Telegraph, 26 May 1989

Today Ignatius would top any league table based on cost efficiency. His methods had the simplicity of genius. They were precisely tailored to the needs of the market and they still lie there waiting to be rediscovered by the next generation of fundholders.
Audiomonitor, January 1997

Secrecy, love of

Form of paranoia endemic in the British civil service, British academia, British government, and the reformed NHS.

In a survey published in April 1992 the Campaign for Freedom of Information said that the Department of Health refused to make public responses to its consultation document on the patient's charter, quoting the Official Secrets Act. The Official Secrets Act 1989 applies to defence, security, law enforcement, and international relations.

Naomi Craft. *BMJ*, 17 December 1994

The government proposes to make all regional directors of public health and directors of research and development into civil servants. In the past, regional directors of public health have been NHS employees who have a right to speak freely in public on behalf of their populations.

Ibid

Selective memory

Sound basis for strongly held opinions.

Seeing an example of bad driving, a man of a certain temperament will remark on it and remember it only if the car is driven by a woman—and thus he convinces himself of women's lesser skill without realising his own errors of judgment.

P B Medawar.
Advice to a Young Scientist, Harper and Row, 1979

Self denial

Reinforcement conditioning for masochists.

I forget who it was recommended men for their soul's good to do each day two things they disliked...it is a precept that I have followed scrupulously; for every day I have got up and I have gone to bed.

W Somerset Maugham.
The Moon and Sixpence, Heinemann, 1919

Self examination

Form of inspection that politicians recommend for the rest of us.

Many of you were intrigued by the way the junior health

minister announced that he was considering a prostatic cancer screening campaign. "The important thing", said Tom Sackville, "Is for men to examine themselves regularly and to see their doctor immediately if they notice any unexplained changes".

I won't go into the sordid details of the ways you suggested Mr Sackville might examine himself. The only point on which you were unanimous was that he should set an example with a public demonstration.

Medical Monitor, 23 August 1995

Sex education

Subversive activity designed to encourage promiscuity, the spread of disease, and the destruction of civilisation as some would like to know it.

Overheard during an American phone-in programme: "These people claim that sex education in schools causes promiscuity. If you have the knowledge, they say, you use it. Heck, I took algebra. Yet I never do maths".

Anecdotal evidence. *Healthcare Management*, June 1995

In the 1940s, the only information on offer about sexually transmitted disease was a list of "VD clinics" posted by the London County Council on the inner walls of public conveniences.

One evening a music hall performer, who earned his living as a *siffleur*, entered what was called "the special department" at the Old Charing Cross Hospital, still wearing the clothes he used in his act: white tie, tails, top hat, and white gloves. He doffed his topper to the receptionist and announced in carefully modulated tones: "I've come in answer to your advertisement in the gentlemen's lavatory in Leicester Square".

Anecdotal evidence. *Healthcare Management*, May 1993

Shaving

Commonest surgical operation performed in Britain. Self mutilation undertaken by men without benefit of protocol or training, using a surgical blade honed to the highest degree of sharpness that technology can provide.

> My investigations reveal that these dangerous surgical
> instruments are freely available in High Street shops where
> they are sold to teenagers who use them with not a hint of
> training, not even a book of instructions. And many bear the
> scars to prove it.
> We've grown used to the Department of Health being
> dilatory in such matters but I'm astonished that the issue
> hasn't been taken up by the Royal College of Surgeons,
> founded as it was by barbers seeking to protect their trade.
> Here surely is a scandal worthy of a *Panorama* investiga-
> tion, a proliferation of victim support groups, or even, dare
> I say it, an Esther Rantzen Special.
> Anecdotal evidence. *Medical Interface*, December 1996

Shirley Williams ploy

Invaluable technique for dealing with garrulous speakers at
medical meetings.

> In the section on chairmanship, I learned how Shirley
> Williams deals with garrulous speakers. When in the chair,
> she nominates speakers in batches, putting those who need
> restraint first in the list. "First you, Dr Gush, then Mr
> Waffle, then Dr Garrulous, Mrs Sane after that, and finally
> Dr Sensible". The shame of holding up the queue apparently
> curbs even the most insensitive of wafflers.
> Review of Meetings, Meetings by Winston Fletcher in:
> One man's burden. *BMJ*, 16 February 1985

SI

Acronym for "Systeme Infernelle".

Side effects

Insignificant reactions that give patients an excuse to stop taking
drugs that doctors know are good for them.

> My abiding memory of the first press conference on the
> beta-blocker "breakthrough" is the uniformity of expression

on the faces of the male hacks when a distinguished cardiologist told us that one of the new drug's "minor side effects" was impotence.

Medical Monitor, 15 November 1995

Silence

The golden core of consultation.

A young woman once entered the surgery of John Abernethy (1764-1831) and, without a word, held out an injured finger for examination. Abernethy dressed the wound in silence. The woman returned a few days later.
"Better?" asked Abernethy. "Better", said the patient. Subsequent visits were conducted in much the same way. On her last visit the woman held out her finger, now healed.
"Well?" asked Abernethy. "Well", she replied.
"Upon my word, madam", said Abernethy, "You are the most rational woman I have ever met".

W Keddie. *Cyclopedia Literary and Scientific Anecdote*, Columbus, Follet, Foster, 1859

Clinicians know the value of maintaining a long silent pause after getting an answer to a question. The longer the silence lasts, the more the interviewee feels the need to break it by adding a remark. And the remark is usually more revealing than the original answer.

This intolerance of overstretched silence develops at an early age. When my son was 11, I took him to a West End matinee and, in the interval, we had to visit the gents. The tiny room had a two berth urinal where my son stood silently alongside a tall severe looking man who wore a black jacket and pinstriped trousers. As the silence stretched, my son felt the need to say something companionable to someone engaged upon the same manly exercise. Eventually he looked up at the unsmiling person alongside and said: "Cartwright can hit the ceiling".

Anecdotal evidence. *Healthcare Management*, June 1995

Silver Screen Syndrome

Distorted perception of age caused by overexposure to stars in childhood.

One milestone, it seems, will forever lie ahead. My age will never catch up with that of the film actors I saw on the screen at the Gaumont, Doncaster, when I was a boy. It's nearly half a lifetime since I was the age at which Errol Flynn, Cary Grant, Betty Grable, Fred Astaire, Marilyn Monroe, *et al*, made those films yet in my mind they still seem older than me, and I suspect they always will. When the films are repeated on television I can *see* they look half my age yet I *know* I'm in the presence of older persons.

Anecdotal evidence. *Medical Interface*, February 1977

The actors themselves are victims of the distortion. Fred Astaire used to say that, when he reached pensionable age, people would approach him in shops and ask: "Weren't you Fred Astaire?" And James Mason once described how two people stared hard at him in the street before one said to the other: "I tell you. It's James Mason in later life".

Ibid

Sin

Synonym for sex. AIDS is a punishment for homosexual behaviour just as syphilis once was for heterosexual misdemeanour.

To welcome sexually transmitted disease as a punishment holily fitting the crime—as so many have agreed with Bunyan since 1680—is a merciless expression of sanctimonious nonsense. The French surgeon Baron Dupuytren had a more charitable approach.

"Have you been with prostitutes?" he asked.

"No, how could you even think of it?" the patient replied.

"Then they have been with you", said Dupuytren.

Richard Gordon.
The Alarming History of Medicine, Mandarin, 1993

Slashing bureaucracy

Dramatic administrative change Health Ministers claim to achieve by reshuffling **job titles**.

The forthcoming change in classification means that

managers can become nurses again, thus diminishing the
number of managers while showing a rise in the number of
nurses.

Melanie Phillips. *Observer*, 29 January 1995

Slides

Academic credentials. Popular with medical audiences. Many
doctors find it difficult to sleep without them. *See* Expert.

Over the years I think I've endured the full repertoire of
slide misfortune: slides appearing upside down, sideways,
back to front, or being gobbled up by the projector; the
projector itself blowing a bulb, blowing a fuse, falling from
its perch, once indeed bursting into flames.

I even strung together an impromptu narrative to match a
set of someone else's slides left in the projector of a
Lancashire hotel after the previous evening's meeting of a
camera club. I managed the first three without giving the
game away but when the fourth turned out to be a mildly
indecent exposure of a young woman making an unambiguous gesture with a model of the Blackpool Tower, I took
fright and confessed. The medical audience noisily
demanded to see the next slide but when they discovered it
was only a moody shot of the sun setting over Morecombe
Bay, they slipped gently back into the arms of Morpheus.
A sort of vagrancy. *An Insider's Guide to the Games
Doctors Play*, Gollancz, 1986

Overcrowded, illegible, and uninterpretable splodge of data
projected on a screen at a scientific meeting.

Whenever such a slide appears on the screen, learned
sócieties should set off an electronic device, sounding much
like the burglar alarms fitted to cars, because a theft of time
and concentration is about to be committed.

Verna Wright. *Hospital Doctor*, 1993

Smile

Enigmatic facial expression. Occasionally a harbinger of laughter; more often an unconscious reflection of a mood that lies

somewhere on the route from fear to delight.

> An obstetrician at a meeting of the Royal Society of
> Medicine claimed that the source of the smile on the Mona
> Lisa was all too obvious to a member of his trade. It was
> that of a woman who'd just been told she was pregnant.
> A woman in the audience claimed equally emphatically it
> was the smile of a woman who'd just been told she was *not*
> pregnant.
> Anecdotal evidence. *Healthcare Management*, October
> 1993

> The idea of National Dental Health Smile Week is an
> abomination. A smile is far too subtle an expression to be
> annexed by coarse folk like dentists. Can anyone seriously
> suggest that all François Mitterand, to name but *un*, needs to
> give him warmth is a few quids' worth of bridgework?
> The only smile that dentists can influence is that ersatz
> expression favoured by politicians and game show hosts and
> memorably defined by S J Perelman when he said of the
> young Shirley Temple that she had a smile "that could melt
> the glue out of a revolving bookcase".
> Body and soul. *Guardian*, January 1988

Social inequalities in health

Finally banished by the British government in 1996.

> The government doesn't like "inequalities" in health. Even
> the word is banned; "variations" is the acceptable word.
> Richard Smith. Keeping the bad news from the journalists.
> *BMJ*, 4 January 1997

Socialspeak

Language imported into medicine in the 1960s and 1970s by a
group of middle aged nurses and doctors who'd grown tired of the
mundanities of everyday clinical medicine.

> Sane and intelligent doctors, who'd reached what our
> mothers used to call "that dangerous age", embarked on
> passionate affairs with the new language. And like many

who embark on passionate affairs in middle life, they quickly lost all sense of reason and discretion and the arcane vocabulary they created is still inflicted on the young by "educationalists" who should know better.

The toxic effect of language on medicine. *Journal of the Royal College of Physicians of London*, November/December 1995

The individual who is known about by others may or may not know that he is known by them; they in turn may or may not know that he knows or does not know of their knowing about him. Further, while believing that they do not know about him, nonetheless he can never be sure. Also, if he knows they know about him, he must, in some measure at least know about them, but if he does not know that they know about him, he may or may not know about them in regard to other matters.

Erving Goffman. *Stigma: Notes on the Management of Spoiled Identity*. Prentice-Hall, 1963

(Recommended reading for GPs and nurses in 1960s)

A factor of considerable importance in naturalistic social-ization contexts is the timing of punishment. In home situations, punishment is often delayed beyond the comple-tion of the deviant behaviour. Does the timing of the administration of a punishment affect its effectiveness as a means of inhibiting undesirable behavior? Mowrer (1960) has provided a theoretical framework for predicting the effects of the timing of punishment. Each component of a response sequence provides sensory feedback in the form of response-produced kinesthetic and proprioceptive cues.

Ronald A Hoppe, *et al. Early Experiences and the Process of Socialisation*. Academic Press 1970

(Further recommended reading for GPs and nurses in 1973)

Sound

Essential attribute for persons who wish to rise through the medical hierarchy. Reliable. Not too cocky. Not too clever. And free of the two great impediments to preferment: "Too clever by half" and "Too big for his boots". All in all, a **decent chap**.

Specialists

Doctors who assume you have what they treat. As opposed to **generalists** who treat what they assume you have.

Speciesism

Defined by national secretary of the Campaign to Abolish Angling: "We do not discriminate between inflicting pain on an animal, or on a child, or on a fish. To think there is any difference is a sort of speciesism".

> Why draw the line at fish? When will someone speak up on behalf of creatures whose daily slaughter is measured not in tens per hour, or in thousands per year, but in millions per second?
>
> *Monitor Weekly*, 17 August 1994

Why are we so cruel to bacteria ?
Let me ask you, by the way of introduction,
Why it doesn't seem to shock us
That we kill the staphylococcus
By inhibiting its powers of reproduction.
Why should we think bacteria
In any way inferior
Because they're small and singularly plain ?
And are we sure a bite
From a hungry phagocyte
Doesn't cause unnecessary pain ?

Why are we so cruel to bacteria
When kindness always helps to clear the air?
Perhaps the salmonella
Is a friendly little fella
Who is longing for a little loving care.
Each small bacterium
Has a loving dad and mum
And a virus
Should inspire us
Every one.
Yet the poor old spirochete
Who only wants to live and eat
Is murdered 'cos he complicates our fun.

There's no need to be cruel to bacteria

Let's recognise each species has its place.
So the next time that you're ill
Throw away that cruel pill
And die with a smile upon your face.
Looking sideways. *World Medicine*, 4 January 1965

Spin doctor

The specialist most in demand in new style NHS Trust hospitals.

Bedfordshire GPs received this notice from their local hospital.

"Florence Ball Ward transferred to the newly decorated Dean Pollard Ward on June 11. It will no longer be known as Florence Ball but will take the name Dean Pollard".

Maybe the hospital hopes the language will disguise what's really happened. Florence Ball Ward has been closed.
Looking sideways. *Medical Monitor*, 17 July 1992

Ward closure improves hospital care for elderly patients.
Headline in *Salisbury Health News Weekly*, 1995

This month, when the London Ambulance Service withdrew transport previously provided to take blind patients and amputees to hospital, it announced the change in a press handout entitled *Planned Improvements for Patient Transport Services*.
Looking sideways. *Medical Monitor*, 28 September 1990

Draft report February 1995:
The pilot projects represent a poor return for the £56 million spent to date by the NHS Executive.
Final report April 1996 after 14 months' "consideration" by the Department of Health:
There is still much work to do to ensure that integrated systems play a full part in the development of the NHS reforms and that the lessons learned for the NHS as a whole increase the value for money from the £56m which the Executive spent.
National audit office report criticising six computer projects, 1995-6

Split brain syndrome

State of self deception induced by chronic dissembling.

> President Ronald Reagan raised cognitive dissonance to an
> art form. He extolled the family though he was divorced and
> never saw his children or grandchildren. He praised God
> and religion but professed none. He could say and believe
> that he was in a photographic unit accompanying the troops
> liberating concentration camps, when he never left the
> United States during the war.
> Peter E Dans. *The Pharos*, Spring 1991

> When man's fancy gets astride of his reason; when
> imagination is at cuffs with the senses; and common
> understanding, as well as common sense, is kicked out of
> doors; the first proselyte he makes is himself.
> Jonathan Swift. *Tale of a Tub*, 1727

Sponsorship

Television advertising of products banned from television
advertising

> Promoters and televisers of sport are made party to cynical
> and flagrant breaches of the "voluntary agreements" that the
> tobacco industry has signed to restrict the promotion of
> cigarettes. The next time you watch televised sport
> remember that a voluntary agreement bans the display of
> brand names on participants, officials, or equipment likely
> to come within range of the cameras.
> Decent people who administer sport and the arts or who
> take part in sport or in sponsored plays and concerts get
> entangled in a web of conspiracy that also enmeshes the
> BBC and ITA.
> And all to help addict people to a drug that kills.
> Body and soul. *Guardian*, November 1984

Sport

(Obsolete) Inconsequential activities called games; 1950s dream
of underprivileged youths enjoying themselves on Duke of

Edinburgh playing fields.
(Now) Humourless custom-booted aggression acted out on international battlefields.

The clichés of the headlines are the clichés of a war correspondent: "England...shame...disgrace...triumph...horror...vanquished".
And whenever I've been favoured with a post-match drink in a soccer boardroom, the air has been thick with phrases beloved of marketing men who like to show off their aggressive amorality: "Nice guys come last", "Blessed are the meek, for they shall make way for the ruthless".

Executive health.
International Management, November 1988

Thirty years ago one of the pleasures that went with walking my dog through Battersea Park was watching 7 and 8 year old schoolboys playing football. One boy stood between each set of goalposts, blowing on his fingers and shouting "Please sir, can I come out now sir?" and the other 20 chased the ball around the field in a joyful pack like a boxful of clockwork toys that had been wound up and poured on to the pitch.
A few weeks ago, I walked past the same pitch. The boys were no larger but were clearly engaged in a sterner activity than that I witnessed 30 years ago. There were no laughs, few smiles, and certainly no free-for-all chases after the ball. On the touch line three track suited masters shouted the aggressive clichés of our time: "Get stuck in", "Put yourself about", "Make your presence felt". And the boys showed they knew what was expected of them as they kicked and tripped and agonised.
Yet, to my jaundiced old eyes, they seemed to be having a lot less fun than I'd seen their fathers have on the same patch of grass.

One man's burden. *BMJ*, January 8 1983

Spouse

Archaic name for husband or wife. Unacceptable in progressive NHS Trusts.

Yesterday I was a spouse but today I am a "bed partner". Having been married for nearly 25 years I was surprised to learn that I could no longer complete a questionnaire about my wife's sleep pattern as a spouse but only in this new title. The NHS obviously regard me as a bed partner first and a spouse second. My wife has not expressed an opinion as to her order of preferences.

David Dumbleton, Stoke-on-Trent, Staffs.
Letter to *Daily Telegraph*, 11 March 1995

Stable relationships

More common between horses than humans. Can occasionally be based on love; more reliable if based on greed.

When Ferenc Molnar, the Hungarian playwright, was successful and middle aged, he made a trip to America but left his young mistress behind in Budapest. On his return, the gossips of the Budapest coffee houses were eager to offer tales of her infidelity and to list her sexual adventures while he was away. Molnar listened to their tales with a smile, then shrugged his shoulders and said: "With them she sleeps only for love. But for money, she sleeps only with me".

George Mikes.
Coffee Houses of Europe, Andre Deutsch 1983

Statistical variation

Art of using press releases to achieve desired political results.

Rich or poor, life is getting better
Britons, rich and poor alike, are living longer, safer lives than 20 years ago, according to figures out yesterday.
The statistics confound claims from poverty campaigners that more than a quarter of the population faces worsening conditions which can lead to early death.
Left-winger academics and lobbyists have claimed that since 1979 millions have been getting poorer with only the already-rich getting richer.
But the new analysis from Office of National Statistics shows...the vast majority are doing well and don't need welfare.

Steve Doughty. *Daily Mail*, December 1996

On page five [of the Office of National Statistics press

release on which the Daily Mail story is based] we learn that "the mortality rate among men in class I and II decreased by about 35%". Underneath, in a separate section, it says "the mortality rate in class V has decreased by 11 per cent since 1979-80, 1982-83. However, it is slightly higher than it was in 1970-72". In other words, the real story of a widening gap—from a twofold to a threefold differential in mortality between rich and poor in 20 years—is thoroughly buried. This press release might have been written by a government spin doctor.
Richard Smith. Keeping the bad news from the journalists.
BMJ, 4 January 1997

Stethoscope

In the right hands, a safe, useful, and versatile instrument provided the users are not unduly influenced by anything they hear through it. *See* Scruffie's Triangle.

Labelling device

In many parts of this country, if you arrive on a doorstep carrying only a little black bag, you are likely to be greeted effusively and led off to inspect the gas meter, the television set, or the broken washing machine. A stethoscope dangling nonchalantly from a pocket or coiled professionally in the hand may cut the effusiveness of the greeting but saves valuable minutes of embarrassing explanation in the kitchen, sitting room, or cupboard under the stairs.

A stethoscope prominently displayed on the rear shelf of a car may deter traffic wardens and the combination of a professionally urgent stride with effective stethoscope display has been known to help seasoned practitioners to gatecrash exclusive parties, to gain free admission to stately homes and gardens, to escape from night-clubs raided by the police, and to bypass suspicious landladies who obstruct the route to young ladies' bedrooms.

Looking sideways. *World Medicine*, June 18 1968

Aid to meditation

Place one end of the instrument on any part of the patient that's handy, use the other ends to plug your external auditory meati, and you create an ambience ideal for reflecting on routine problems like "What is the matter with this patient?" and more important ones like "What is his name?" or "What crisp, reassuring, non-discussion-provoking phrase will allow me to get out of this room and home in time to see the football on television?"

Sophisticated practitioners often improve the thought-enhancing qualities of their stethoscopes by keeping the earpieces permanently bunged with cotton wool thus eliminating distracting sounds that may intrude if the instrument is placed inadvertently over the heart or other noisy organ.

The sound-proofed instrument is particularly useful for dealing with talkative patients whom you can halt in full flow by applying the instrument to their chests and telling them to breathe deeply.

Anecdotal evidence. *Healthcare Management*, March 1995

Stiff upper lip

Side effect of diet high in moral fibre. Usually associated with stiffening of backbone.

Straight face

Essential component of a solemn consultation

Dr John Davies of Kirby in Cleveland points out that at no stage in their tutelage are aspiring GPs taught how to cope with that dreaded moment in a solemn consultation when a patient, wholly oblivious of the import of the words being uttered, says something that threatens to "corpse" the GP. Dr Davies illustrates the need for training by quoting two patients who attended within a week. Both were men complaining of impotence.

The first said he'd had the problem for some time and had finally summoned up the courage to visit the doctor "to get himself straightened out". The second, a man in his 60s, wasn't sure whether problem was normal for his age because he "didn't have a yardstick to measure it by".

In both instances Dr Davies managed to survive by reaching for his handkerchief and pretending to blow his nose but he fears this traditional technique may one day prove inadequate.

Monitor Weekly, 12 April 1995

Straight man

Phrase borrowed from the variety stage to describe the primary duty of a junior hospital doctor.

He must provide suitable entries for one of the half dozen humorous stories in his chief's repertoire and give a dutiful laugh at the right moment so as to lead in the congregation. Tedious as the role may be, it is worse for the registrar and worse still for the ward sister, both of whom have heard the stories many more times than the houseman. Have you noticed how registrars go to imaginary telephone calls, and sisters unaccountably go and take somebody's temperature at certain moments during the chief's round ? Perhaps you can understand it now.
Richard Asher. Medical salesmanship,
Middlesex Hospital Medical Journal, February 1960

Student

A subversive.

Someone who thinks otherwise. It is dangerous to treat this healthy state of mind.
Richard L Day. Quoted by William A Silverman in: *Human Experimentation: A Guided Step into the Unknown,*
Oxford University Press, 1985

Surgical spirit

Verve shown by surgeons when protecting their craft from invasion by women.

As a female surgeon I can only despair at my own specialty, orthopaedics, where women represent less than 2% of consultants and around 3% of trainees. This is probably the worst record among the major specialties for the recruitment and training of women in hospital medicine.

My own experiences as a trainee would hardly encourage other members of my sex. The worst episode occurred in 1991, when I was a career registrar in Scotland expecting my first child, and my professor informed me that I would not be regarded as a "doctor in training" for the purposes of maternity employment rights. I received my P45 in the post. After a lengthy appeal I was reinstated and completed my registrar rotation. When I returned to work I was not made welcome and no apology was forthcoming.

Sian Caich. Letter to *BMJ*, 3 June 1995

Sycophantic

Traditional attitude towards seniors adopted by those who seek advancement in the medical profession. Not always effective.

The ambitious make too obvious a point of being polite to those who can promote their interests and are proportionately uncivil to those who cannot. "I hope we don't have to be nice to him", an ambitious young Oxford don said to me of a kindly old buffer with an amateurish interest in science who was dining at High Table. He wasn't, and although this particular episode did not harm him, it was symptomatic of a state of mind that did.

P B Medawar.
Advice to a Young Scientist, Harper and Row, 1979

Bankers, it seems, have caught up with a truth already known to generations of junior doctors. Sucking up to the boss is good for you. John D Watt, of Kansas State University, describes in the *Journal of Psychology* how he subjected 108 bank employees to a personality test designed to measure sycophancy. The "yes men" were more likely to be promoted, to earn the approval of their superiors, and to get "positive" assessment reports. Juniors who indulged in high levels of ingratiating behaviour won high marks for "co-operation, competence, motivation, promotion potential, and overall performance".

Medical Monitor, 6 October 1993

The sycophantic conventions of our own profession are well defined—most memorably, in my experience, by John Forrest Smith, who was a paediatrician at St Thomas's when I was a student. When he learned that a final year student had become engaged to the daughter of another St Thomas's consultant, he remarked: "How odd. Doesn't he know that the traditional route to advancement in this hospital is PR not PV".

Ibid

Syndrome

Random collection of quirks and oddities that, if given a name, will be readily diagnosed by doctors who will then think they've achieved something.

> Luposlipaphobia: The fear of being pursued by timber wolves around a kitchen table while wearing socks on a newly waxed floor.
> Gary Larson. Quoted in *Monitor Weekly*, 26 May 1993

Syntactical perseveration

Communication disorder that leads people to choose words that impose their own meaning on a sentence.

> Sister Shirley competes for the Nurse of the Year title. She says: "The hospital's ambulance men entered me without my knowing".
> *Ilford Hospital Newsletter*, 1974

> I have arranged gastroscopy with small bowel biopsy and colonoscopy to be performed at one sitting.
> Letter from gastroenterologist to William Richardson, of
> Houghton-Le-Spring.
> Quoted in *Monitor Weekly*, 7 April 1994

> In October 1996, Avon Health Authority organised "a unique training programme" for practice nurses entitled "The ins and outs of sex".
> The chosen venue was the Bristol Society for the Blind.
> *Medical Monitor*, 8 January 1997

Terminate

Originally **Decorated Municipal Gothic** for "stop" but addictive use has broadened its meaning to the point of ambiguity. *See* Visualise.

> A GP friend received this note from a psychiatrist who'd been looking after one of his patients: "She was an intelligent, co-operative, well motivated person and would have been offered further treatment but she terminated herself".
>
> Assuming she'd committed suicide, my friend telephoned to find out what had happened. He was told rather frostily that his patient had stopped treatment of her own accord. "If you bother to look through your correspondence", said the psychiatrist, "You'll find that we sent you a note".
>
> At which point my friend terminated the conversation. He found it more difficult, he says, to terminate his urge to terminate the psychiatrist.
>
> *Medical Monitor*, 2 April 1997

Third Law of Human Perversity

Form of blindness that afflicts the deeply committed. If a medical editor publishes opinions from opposite sides of a vigorously contested argument, each side will protest that the journal is biased and will assume that the editor's personal views coincide with those of their opponents.

> The faithful, it seems, rarely read articles with which they agree—maybe they find them too boring—but they devote assiduous attention to any article that angers them, as if they need a regular fix of self righteousness to sustain their beliefs. As an ex-editor, I am still, 10 years later, credited with a portfolio of beliefs that are wholly incompatible.
>
> World Medicine. A sort of obituary. *BMJ*, 3 October 1990

Throughput

Managerial measure of efficient use of hospital beds.

> Mrs Singh of Doncaster went into hospital to have her

varicose veins done. On coming round from the anaesthetic she unwisely got up and went to the loo. When she came back four minutes later somebody else had been given her bed.

David Delvin. *BMA News Review*, 10 May 1995

Tittivulation

Interpretative disorder endemic in departments that concern themselves with "health care delivery systems".

Named after Tittivulus, a minor demon who appears in Michael Ayrton's *The Verbiage Collector* and is given the task of collecting in sacks the world's "negligences, pomposities, and vanities of utterance".

As evidence of Tittivulus's current workload, Dr Hilary Graver offers an article from King's Healthcare Trust's *GP News* describing how the trust has "taken on the task over the next two to three years of radically transforming the way in which healthcare services are delivered". It hopes to fulfil this modest ambition through a technique called Re-engineering which "differs from all other quality initiatives by being a radical and total system".

If you seek examples of Ayrton's "vanities of utterance", try these three.

- "Re-engineering is the rethinking and redesign of a whole health care delivery system to achieve an order of improvement in performance which cannot be achieved incrementally or parochially".
- "Re-engineering is customer focused, top driven and involves the whole organisation".
- "At the end of the programme, King's Healthcare's delivery systems should be more accessible, simpler and faster and more value should be passed on to the customer. Front end investment is required however and King's has already established a Team to take the programme forward".

Seasoned verbiage collectors might conclude that the need is not so much for front end investment as for rear end disposal.

Monitor Weekly, 7 September 1994

Tonsils and adenoids

Lumps of lymphoid tissue that exist only to provide food, clothes, and private education for the children of ear, nose, and throat surgeons.

Top doctor (Hackspeak)

Any doctor a journalist finds at home and willing to give a "quote" close to a deadline.

Total Allergy Syndrome

Dramatic illness diagnosed in the early 1980s amid great publicity, including television pictures of young women gulping oxygen and living in plastic tents to protect them from the dreaded allergens. Solemn "experts" told us that the most seriously afflicted were, in effect, "allergic to the 20th century" and kindly folk raised money to send them to specialised clinics that would save their lives.

> What has happened to the people who made the diagnosis? I remember upsetting some of our complementary colleagues at the time by writing in *Punch* about a GP who'd become afflicted. He'd started with the simple everyday diseases of general practice: occasional allergy to the BMA, certain patients, and the chairman of his FPC (remember those?). But these symptoms failed to run their normal fluctuating course and were soon transcended by more serious allergies: to repeat prescriptions, postgraduate tutors, and particularly the Royal College of General Practitioners.
> A perceptive partner diagnosed him as suffering from total allergy to 20th century general practice and sympathetic colleagues raised money to build him a patient-proof bungalow just outside Frinton.
> He emerged only last year and, as an expression of gratitude, used a legacy to convert a country house into a safe haven for victims of the latest outbreak—GPs with total allergy to the internal market. He could be busy.
> *Medical Monitor*, 19 February 1997

Touch base

Trustspeak imperative. Leave a message on my answering machine

Toxicology

A way of exterminating rodents rather then people. Hence its unpopularity with animal liberationists.

Traditional British diet

Phrase used by food manufacturers seeking to defend eating habits criticised by the **health lobby.**

> The phrase evokes an image of Essex and Elizabeth exchanging wicked glances over platefuls of baked beans, sausages, and fatty chips, and hints that the glory that blazed at Agincourt, Blenheim, and Waterloo was won by yeomen with knapsacks stuffed with packets of crisps, chocolate bars, and bottles of brown sauce.
>   One man's burden. *BMJ*, 31 August 1985

Training

A way, some would have us believe, of turning a sow's ear into a silk purse. Not to be confused with **education.**

> Most of the complaints I hear from patients are not about the doctor's intellectual failing but about a lack of some human quality like understanding or sympathy. Some individuals seem incapable of developing these qualities to the level that a doctor needs and I can't accept that you can always correct that defect by "training" everyone in Communication or Empathy. Unless individuals have a real interest in the bizarre ways in which other people can live their lives, they may be impervious to training in certain human skills.
>   To believe otherwise is to accept that Claudio Abbado can say to the leader of the London Symphony Orchestra: "We sound a bit thin on the strings these days, Charlie. Just nip

down the pub, like a good boy, and pick out a few likely lads. We just need to send them on a violin training course to get us back on top of the charts".

One man's burden. *BMJ*, 13 April 1985

Tonight's speaker is a senior officer of the Royal College of Nursing and she has been talking about training. When she finishes one of the nurses in the audience tells the story of how she had suddenly found herself confronted by a man who had lost his entire family in a road accident. The burden of the speaker's response to this is that no nurse could cope with such a situation without a training in psychology. I can't resist putting in my oar:

"What worries me is that saying that sort of thing will make people think that they shouldn't even try to help unless they have specialised training. Some people can do these things and some people can't, the main qualification they need is experience of life".

She looks impatient with me and I go on.

"Don't you think it is possible that going on a course in psychology might actually make somebody worse at helping in this situation?"

She does not.

"Don't you think there must be some examples of training courses which are counterproductive?"

No, she does not. Training is training. By definition, it is a good thing. Like love or happiness.

James Willis. *The Paradox of Progress*,
Radcliffe Medical Press, 1995

Transcultural medicine

1. Intractable problem facing a doctor trained south of Watford trying to do a locum in Tyneside.
2. The complexities of treating people in a multiethnic society.

Mr H K Basu, an Indian graduate who is a consultant gynaecologist in Gravesend, was consulted by a Punjabi woman. Because he doesn't speak the language he asked his house surgeon, who does, to take the history. The history taking started with a lot of giggling and, when Mr Basu asked what was going on, the house surgeon explained that the woman had asked: "If your boss can't speak Punjabi, what is he doing in Gravesend?"

Monitor Weekly, 28 August 1992

Trivial illness

An illness suffered by someone else.

Trolley

Outmoded name for new improved NHS bed. Acceptance of the new nomenclature could dramatically reduce waiting times for admission.

> There is no difference between a trolley and a bed. Both have wheels, both have sides to prevent you falling out, both can be bent in the middle and both give you back ache. All that is required is a stock of small labels reading *This is not a trolley, it is a bed* and one can be popped on each item after a patient has been lying on it for more than, say, two hours.
> John Townend. *BMA News Review*, 11 December 1996

Trust

Paradoxical title given to NHS management units that inspire little confidence in their employees. *See* mistrust, distrust.

Trustspeak

Language used by medical administrators who think it endows them with the correct macho image for the post-Thatcher age. Described by Michael Leapman in the *Observer* (January 1993) as "Verbal detritus bred from the half-digested nostrums of the business schools and the self-important hype of the public relations industry".

> You need to be aware that effective 9.00 am on 13th December, the Executive Board has agreed that a "ring-fence" shall apply to the bed envelope of each general management grouping across the hospital. Thus the intention is that the Medical grouping, the Surgical grouping and Specialist service grouping for example will consume their

own smoke in meeting bed requirements.
> *Joint memorandum from chief executive and medical director*, Addenbrooke's NHS Trust, Cambridge 1993

The planning process will consider the volume of each critical resource consumed by each episode and will produce load plans by specialty over an appropriate horizon. It will then aggregate these upwards into an overall resource plan so that capacity and production levels can be set to meet the level of demand.
> Mick Bolton. New look for medical administration.
> *Synapse, The Journal for Medical Staff at East Surrey Hospital*, 1995

NHSME guidance dictates that a purchaser is within its rights to refuse to pay for a patient's treatment if prior authorisation for non-emergency referrals, other than tertiary referrals, is not obtained before either notifying the patient of treatment commencement dates or undertaking treatment itself.

It is this authority's intention to strictly enforce this guidance with effect from 2 August 1993 for all non-emergency referrals other than tertiary referrals (including all relevant outpatient attendances both new and follow up).
> *Notice from chief executive of an authority that chooses to call itself Health in Leicestershire*

The primary function of Facilities Management (FM) is to enable the organisation to plan and develop its business strategy, whilst operationally, FM services can be delivered through a range of "mixed economies" to total outsourcing.
> *Information circulated to GPs by Essex Rivers Healthcare Trust*, 1997

Truth

What little is left after rigorous elimination.

It is virtually hopeless to try to prove that anything is true; disproof on the other hand may be completely decisive.
> Karl Popper. *The Logic of Scientific Discovery*,
> Routledge and Kegan Paul, 1954

Type O virus

Computers are not the only inanimate objects to suffer virus infection. Dictating machines and typewriters, if left uncovered in medical surroundings, can be invaded by the type O organism that penetrates their DNA and subtly distorts the words they produce. The infection produces a variety of symptoms:

Illuminating homophone

> He is opening his bowels twelve times daily and is going through a toilet role a day.
>
> *Letter signed and posted by Dr Marcus Wilde*
> *of Loughborough*

> Contraceptive pills are not suiting her and other methods make her soar.
>
> *Letter found in patient's notes by Dr Kiaran O'Sullivan*
> *of Northwich*

Image enhancement

> The typewriter possessed by Judy Gosney, a GP in Spalding, produced the sentence: "The tonsils are small and scared and barely visible behind the tonsillar pillars". Here the kindly type O virus transmutes those nasty scarred tonsils into sympathetic creatures cowering behind pillars to hide from the surgeon's knife.
>
> *Monitor Weekly,* 30 November 1994

> Thank you for sending this woman along. I have started the bull rolling by requesting a semen analysis.
>
> *Letter from Hertfordshire infertility clinic*

Freudian

> We had an expensive discussion of his symptoms.
>
> *Letter from consultant to Dr Anthony Abrahams of Oxford*

Distorting spacebar

> Today I have aspirated the knee under a septic technique.
>
> *Letter to Dr J A Ball of Birmingham*

197

Typical

As described in textbooks. Therefore often used in medicine as synonym for untypical.

> In my student days, a surgical registrar called to see a patient in casualty told us: "We must admit this chap for the firm to see. He shows the typical picture and we don't see that very often".
> The toxic effect of language on medicine. *Journal of the Royal College of Physicians of London*, November/December 1995

> Take, for example, Pel-Ebstein fever. Every student and every doctor knows that cases of Hodgkin's disease may show a fever that is high for one week and low for the next week, and so on. Does this phenomenon really exist at all? If you collect the charts of 50 cases of Hodgkin's disease and compare them with the charts of 50 cases of disseminated malignant fever, do you really believe you could pick out even one or two cases because of the characteristic fever? I think it is very unlikely indeed. Yet if, by the vagaries of chance, one case of Hodgkin's did run such a temperature, the news would soon travel round. "There's a good case of Hodgkin's disease in Galen Ward. You ought to have a look. It shows the typical Pel-Ebstein fever very well".
> Richard Asher. *Richard Asher Talking Sense*, Pitman Medical, 1972

Uncooperative patient

One who is impervious to simple straightforward explanation.

> *From a letter written by a surgeon about a 73 year old stroke victim:*
> I explained that surgery carries a 4% risk of stroke, and that after surgery her risk of stroke is about $1\frac{1}{2}\%$ per year. This will give her a 5 year stroke risk of about 10%. I have explained that best medical treatment carries about an 11%

risk of stroke in the next year and about 7% risk of stroke every year after that. This would give her a 5 year stroke risk of about 40%. I have also advised them of the nature of carotid surgery and the recovery expected.
I am afraid she seemed a little bewildered and taken aback by my explanations.

Dr R S Smith, GP in Helston, Cornwall.
Personal communication

Understanding

What people seek when they write to one another, except when they write a **scientific paper**.

We need to rediscover a language in which we can express our ideas about medicine in a clear and interesting way. What is good enough for novelists and philosophers ought to be good enough for doctors,
Open day lecture. *Royal College of Physicians of London*,
July, 1995

I see but one rule: to be clear. If I am not clear, all my work crumbles to nothing.
Stendahl, in a letter to Balzac. Quoted in *Writers on Writing*.
Phoenix House 1948

I write as I walk because I want to get somewhere; and I write as straight as I can, just as I walk as straight as I can, because that is the best way to get there.
H G Wells. *Experiment in Autobiography*, Gollancz, 1934

What can be said at all can be said clearly, and what we cannot talk about we must pass over in silence.
Ludwig Wittgenstein. Preface, *Tractatus Logico-Philosophicus*, 1922. Reissued by Routledge and Kegan Paul, 1949

Uninformed fears

Affective disorder induced by media reports about medicine.

You asked that, in dealing with public attitudes, I should "try particularly to distinguish justifiable anxieties from

199

uninformed fears". The only distinction I can make is that uninformed fears are what patients suffer before doctors tell them what they are going to do to them and justifiable anxieties are what they suffer after they've been told. The demands of public opinion. Constraints on the Advance of Medicine.

Proceedings Royal Society of Medicine, December 1974

Unprecedented (Trustspeak)

Adjective used to describe emergency admissions every January.

Unsatisfactory patient

One whose illness fails to respond to the skills of a well trained doctor.

Value for money

1. Cheap.
2. A judgment the NHS entrusts to those known to have little sense of value.

Victory for commonsense (BMAspeak)

Unworkable compromise.

Village cricket

Traditional sport of rural general practitioners. Presence on village green gives appearance of availability while deterring interruption.

Dr W G Grace never left the crease no matter how grave the

summons. Even umpires found it difficult to dislodge him. Once when he was leaving his house carrying a cricket bag an anxious young woman accosted him. "I think my twins have got measles", she said. "Can you come?"
"Not just now", replied the doctor. "But contact me at the ground if their temperatures reach 206 for two".
Looking sideways. *Medical Monitor*, 14 September 1990

Visualise

Originally **Decorated Municipal Gothic** for "foresee". Used since the 1950s as verbal seasoning to add "scientific" flavour to any medical statement to do with "viewing" or "seeing". *See* Terminate.

I visualise the need for further examinations to enable us to visualise the exact position of this foreign body.
Henry Gillespie.
X Ray report, St Peter's Hospital, Chertsey, 1963

Vocation

Mystical influence that guides people towards a medical career.

As a local GP he was recruited to help out at a careers night at the school.
"So you're thinking about becoming a doctor", he said to the teenage boy
"Yes".
"Which branch of medicine do you do you think you might be interested in?"
"Private", said his mother.
Looking sideways. *Medical Monitor*, 27 March 1992

Waiting lists

Provisional
A form of psychotherapy. Random numbers assembled by civil

servants in Department of Health to engender **feel good factor** in their Ministers.

Actual

Technical data of little public interest.

> The Department of Health has failed to publicise the latest waiting list figures which reveal the number of people waiting for inpatient treatment last September reached 1 071 101, the highest total since records began. The department's decision to bury the news of the statistics contrasts sharply with the trumpeting by ministers of the "provisional" figures for that same period, published last November, which showed a slight drop in the number of patients waiting in the previous quarter to June.
>
> A spokesman said it was decided the figures were "not newsworthy".
>
> *Independent*, 25 January 1995

Waiting to happen (Hackspeak)

A limbo where accidents linger for a time before being set free.

> A man had fallen off a hospital trolley and broken his hip. At lunch time a television news reader interrogated one of the hospital's surgeons who was determined to give a mundane explanation. Irritated, the news reader sought to add urgency: "Wouldn't you say, doctor, that this was an accident waiting to happen?" The surgeon, God bless him, replied: "Er...no".
>
> Later the news reader wound up the bulletin: "And on this programme a member of the medical staff denied that this was an accident waiting to happen", thus giving the incident a roundness of zen-like perfection. It was as if the Rev Ian Paisley had walked out of a negotiation and said: "It's all over bar the shouting".
>
> Looking sideways. *Medical Monitor*, 25 September 1992

Wasting

What happens to resources when the NHS dabbles in computers.

> In 1993 the House of Commons public accounts committee

condemned the waste of £20 million of NHS money on the Wessex computer project.

In 1996 Alan Langlands, the NHS chief executive, appeared before the committee to explain how, to achieve a saving of £3.4 million, the NHS had spent £106 million on six hospital information support systems. He was questioned by the MP for Swansea.

Alan Williams: If you saw someone walk into a brick wall, pick himself up and walk into that brick wall again, would the thought perhaps cross your mind that he might be either drunk or of unsound mind?

Alan Langlands: Yes.

Alan Williams: That is exactly what you did...You have blundered in and lost another £106 million.

Footnotes. *Private Eye*, 24 January 1997

We

Impersonal pronoun favoured by doctors. Can be used not just to patronise patients—"And how are we today?"—but to absolve the speaker from personal responsibility:

"We'll take you into hospital".
"We'll get rid of that lump for you".
"We did our best but Nature took its course".

Well known

Often used in medicine, as in politics, as a synonym for true. A sceptic shudders at any statement that begins: "It is a well known fact that...".

> The result of self abuse is always—mind you, always—that the boy after a time becomes weak and nervous and shy, he gets headaches and probably palpitations of the heart, and if he carries on too far he very often goes out of his mind and becomes an idiot. *It is a well known fact that* a large number of the lunatics in our asylums have made themselves mad by indulging in this vice although at one time they were sensible, cheery boys like any one of you.
>
> Baden-Powell.
> *Scouting for Boys*, Boy Scout Association, 1908

Dr X says it is well known that anorexia, weight loss and vomiting are uncommon in pernicious anaemia. He is right. It is well known. The error in his argument is that he has assumed that what is well known (that is, generally accepted) is therefore true.

Richard Asher. Letter to *BMJ*, 1961

Wisdom

The valuable nugget that lies buried somewhere in every discovery.

We should be careful to get out of an experience only the wisdom that is in it—and stop there; lest we be like the cat that sits down on a hot stove-lid. She will never sit on a hot stove-lid again, and that is well; but also she will never sit down on a cold one any more.

Mark Twain. *Pudd'nhead Wilson's New Calendar, Following the Equator*, Viking Press, 1896 [Written in Guildford]

Working out

Extravagant forms of exercise undertaken not for pleasure but to improve "body image".

The beneficial effects of the regular quarter-hour's exercise before breakfast is more than offset by the mental wear and tear in getting out of bed 15 minutes earlier.

Simeon Strunsky.
Quoted in *Medical Monitor*, 8 January 1997

Workshop (Trustspeak)

Talkshop.

Writing up results

Paradoxical phrase used by medical scientists when writing down results.

Wrong word malapropism

Self defining condition first described by Kingsley Amis.
Common occurrence in general practice.

> Doctor, my bowels have become erotic.
> *Elderly patient speaking to Dr A N Hill of Holt in Norfolk.*
>
> I've just put in for my infidelity allowance.
> *Patient of Eric Webb of Milton Keynes*
>
> I've brought the baby to be humanised.
> I've had two servile smears.
> I can't conceive. I've been serialised.
> My daughter's just had a baby. The hospital asked me to
> bring her to the doctor for a postmortem.
> Tom Madden.
> General practice notes from the 1950s and '60s. Quoted in
> *Medical Monitor*, 22 January and 5 February 1997

―――――

Xmas

Season when doctors are encouraged to share the festive spirit.

> One thing that never ceased to amaze me at Christmas was
> the procession of patients bringing presents to my door. The
> value of the present always related inversely to the service
> I'd rendered; the nearer I'd come to actually killing
> someone, the more flamboyant the acknowledgement. That
> shouldn't have surprised me because there's nothing like
> making a mistake to render a GP dedicatedly attentive. As
> we desperately try to repair the damage we've done we grow
> lavish with our time and our concern, and the punters
> interpret our hyperactivity as an expression of loving care.
> It was a sobering moment—if you know what I mean—
> when I realised that my clinical incompetence kept my
> family in booze for at least six months every year.
> *Medical Monitor*, December 21 1995

> At 4 am on Christmas Day, 1981, Dr H K Gooding was

roused from a deep sleep by a 'phone call from the night sister at Surbiton Hospital. One of his patients who had severe cor pulmonale had climbed out of his cot, wandered into an empty office, telephoned 999, and ordered not just an ambulance but a mountain rescue team and a St Bernard dog before returning to his cot and falling asleep.

The ambulance service, suspecting a medical jape, rang the sister to complain but she made a shrewder diagnosis of the source. When Dr Gooding arrived, he found his patient calm and friendly. The good doctor explained he'd been unable to get hold of a mountain rescue team but that he himself was a St Bernard. Whereupon his patient asked him to give him some brandy.

Dr G said he was fresh out of brandy, but suggested a small injection might help. He then administered 5 ml diazepam intravenously—a traditional GP way of saying: "God rest you, merry gentleman".

World Medicine, 9 January 1982

X Ray Vision

Form of tunnel vision specific to radiologists. The result of long hours spent in dark rooms looking at negatives.

Yellow streak

Superficial skin discolouration over spinal column signifying lack of moral fibre in diet.

Yorkshire relish

Delight provoked in those who live in the Ridings by the antics of those who don't.

In the early 1970s, the Yorkshire Post ran a series of stories chronicling the progress of a party of 20 Japanese chicken sexers who were visiting the county to share their skills with local farmers.

A friend of mine then practising in a small Yorkshire town claims that one morning as he crossed the bridge at his local railway station he saw one of the porters gazing down on the visitors bunched on a platform below. As the GP approached, the porter turned and said: "They may be bloody clever these Japanese, doctor, but they don't know the right platform for Sowerby Bridge".

Medical Monitor, 28 April 1993

An inner city GP spent a week walking in the Yorkshire Dales. As lunch time approached on the first day, he passed a Dalesman repairing a stone wall and stopped to ask the way to the nearest pub. Without speaking, the Dalesman pointed along the road in the direction the GP was already travelling.

"How long will it take?" asked the GP.

"Dunno", said the Dalesman without looking up.

The doctor shrugged and walked on muttering curses on Yorkshire and its inhabitants. When he was 100 yards down the road, he heard the Dalesman shout. He stopped and turned and the Dalesman repeated the shout: "About 11 minutes". The GP, hot and tired, shouted back: "Why the hell didn't you tell me that when I first asked you?"

The Dalesman looked surprised and a little hurt. "No need to speak to me like that", he said. "I hadn't seen you walk, had I?"

Monitor Weekly, 18 May 1994

Youth

A state of mind. Systematically eliminated from the medical life cycle.

The kids we bring into medical school are wonderful, with the highest possible qualities. We then submerge them in facts and beat the imagination out of them.

Kenneth Calman. *Utopia and Other Destinations*, BBC Radio 4, 29 March 1997

From the earliest times the old have rubbed it into the young that they are wiser than they, and before the young had discovered what nonsense this was they were old too, and it profited them to carry on the imposture.

W Somerset Maugham. *Cakes and Ale*, Heinemann, 1930

Zeal

Essential yet dangerous component of medical practice.

In an ideal world radical treatment would be given only by conservative doctors and conservative treatment only by radical ones. Then the doctor's attitude would always work in the patient's favour.

In my experience it's not the pioneers in medicine, but their acolytes, who are prone to uncritical enthusiasm. They are the ones who need to be reminded of the notice that William Silverman devised for the wall of a fireworks factory: "It is better to curse the darkness than to light the wrong candle".

Medical Monitor, 30 April 1997

Zero option (Trustspeak)

The role of altruism in an internal market.

Soundings

From BMJ columnists

Edited by Ruth Holland

Doctors as ideal party guests . . . being propositioned by a patient . . . making your own gunpowder . . . appointments committees . . . hospital architecture . . . breast implants . . . trees . . . the royal touch . . .

Each week in the *BMJ* the regular columnists of the "Soundings" page – two general practitioners, three hospital doctors, three journalists – expound wittily, passionately, or forcefully on matters relating to medicine and the world at large. This selection brings together a choice of contributions from a year's "Soundings" by Trisha Greenhalgh, Julie Welch, Bernard Dixon, Colin Douglas, James Owen Drife, George Dunea, Tony Smith, and David Widgery.

Highly personal and eloquently expressed, these opinion pieces will entertain, inform, and exasperate you by turns.

ISBN 0-7279-0776 X
89 pages